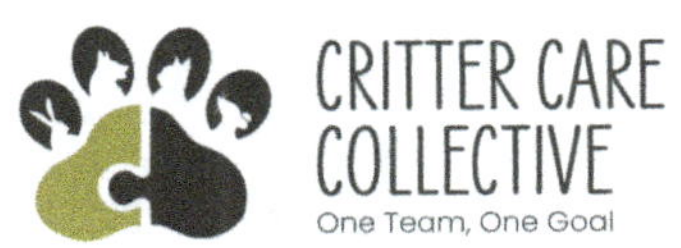

THE CAT OWNER'S GUIDE TO HEALTH EMERGENCIES

Essential Tips to Recognize, Respond, and Prepare for Cat Emergencies

Dr. Gal Chivvis

Critter Care Collective, LLC

Printed in the United States of America
ISBN: 978-1-967320-00-4 (paperback)
ISBN: 978-1-967320-01-1 (Ebook)
Library of Congress Control Number: 2026903071

Written by Dr. Gal Chiwis, DVM
Cover and interior design by Dr. Gal Chivvis
Editing and Proofing: Wendy Reed
Professional Consult: Cristine Hayes, DVM, DABT, DABVT

First printing 2026

Business Address:
5000 Thayer Center
STE C
Oakland, MD 21550

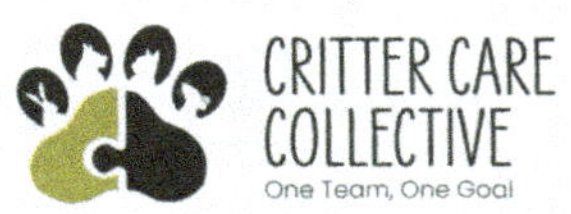

MY CAT'S NAME:

____

My local veterinarian's name,
phone number, and address:

____

____

____

Emergency veterinarian contact
information:

____

____

____

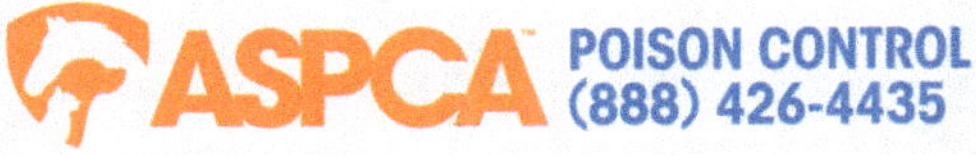

A Note to Cat Families

As a loving pet owner, your primary goal is to ensure your cat remains happy and healthy. However, emergencies can arise unexpectedly. Knowing when to act quickly can be crucial to your cat's wellbeing and may even save your cat's life. In this book, I'll help you distinguish between minor issues and true emergencies, and I'll highlight warning signs that require immediate attention.

Keep in mind that these are general guidelines only. Some emergencies can be difficult to recognize and may not present with classic signs. Ultimately, you know your cat best, so if you have concerns, please reach out to a veterinarian.

Before we begin, let's get some things out of the way.

DISCLAIMER

I created this book to educate pet owners because I believe the best care happens when pet families and veterinary professionals work together as a team.

The information in this book is based on my experience as an emergency veterinarian and is intended for educational purposes only. It does not provide a diagnosis or replace veterinary care. Veterinary approaches may vary, and my recommendations may differ from those of your veterinarian. Always follow the advice of the veterinarian who can examine your cat and knows them best.

Let us begin going through information about emergencies! I recommend you take the time to read through this book BEFORE any emergencies should strike so that you will be prepared. I will do my best to provide recommendations and suggestions for practical tools to help along the way!

What is Your Emergency Toolkit?

Veterinary professionals use a variety of techniques to assess a pet's condition and determine stability. While these skills take years of training to master, there are key observations pet owners can learn to help assess their cat's well-being during an emergency. Recognizing particular signs can help you feel more confident in determining whether you are facing a true emergency.

By observing specific indicators, you can also provide your veterinarian with critical information, allowing for faster and more accurate care.

Remember, if you're ever uncertain, it's always wise to seek professional advice from a veterinarian.

Below, you'll find a quick-reference list of the key indicators in your toolkit and where to find them in the book.

TOOL	SECTION	PAGE #
Resting Respiratory Rate	Difficulty Breathing	110
Urinary Bladder Assessment	Urinary Issues	114
Eye Assessment for Hydration	Vomiting/Diarrhea	133
Gum Moisture Assessment	Vomiting/Diarrhea	133
Capillary Refill Time	Vomiting/Diarrhea	134
Skin Tenting	Vomiting/Diarrhea	135
Pain Scale	Pain/Difficulty Moving	141

You'll find several important handouts throughout the book that are designed to assist you during various stages of your pet's care. Feel free to photocopy or scan these pages for your use.

Additionally, I'm happy to provide these handouts as full-page PDFs for your convenience. You can access them on my website at www.crittercarecollective.com or simply email me at crittercarecollective@gmail.com with the subject line: "Emergency PDFs."

DOCUMENT	PURPOSE	PAGE #
First Aid Supplies Checklist	Emergency Preparation	2
Know Your Local ER Options	Emergency Preparation	4
Medical Decision Authorization Form	Emergency Preparation/ Provide to caretaker if you are away from your cat	7
Sick Visit Information Sheet	Emergency Response/ Prepare for a sick visit to assist your veterinarian and ensure nothing is missed	9

CHAPTERS

Chapter 1:   1
How to Prepare for Emergencies

Chapter 2:   13
10 Most Common Emergencies

Chapter 3:   72
10 Most Common Toxicities

Chapter 4:   106
How to Recognize an Emergency

Chapter 5:   155
Preventing Emergencies

Chapter 6:   172
Emergency Toolkit & Response Flowcharts

HOW TO PREPARE FOR EMERGENCIES

Emergencies can happen without warning, and being prepared can make all the difference when it comes to your cat's health and safety. Having a well-stocked first-aid kit, knowing the location of your nearest emergency veterinary clinic, and maintaining an emergency plan are essential for managing stressful situations effectively.

In this chapter, I'll guide you through building a comprehensive pet emergency kit, planning ahead, and taking steps to ensure you're prepared for the unexpected.

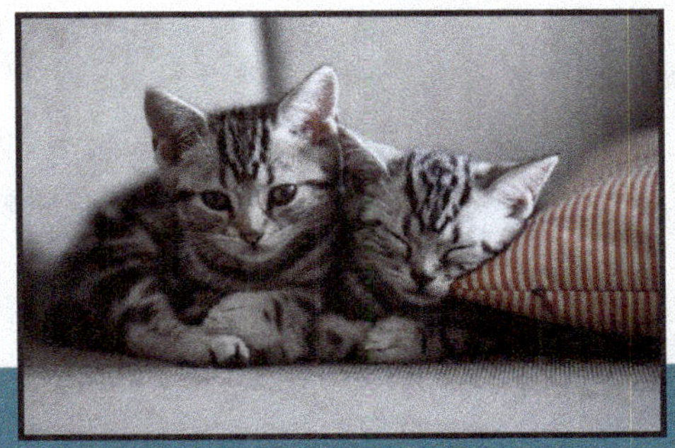

Chapter Highlights:

1. Emergency First Aid Kit Checklist

2. Knowing Your Local ER Options

3. Having an Emergency Plan

4. Preparing Your Cat for Care in Your Absence

5. Key Information for the Veterinarian

6. A Note About CPR

7. Pet Insurance Benefits

A well-equipped first-aid kit is a lifesaver in emergencies. It enables you to address common health issues and injuries right away, giving you peace of mind and the time needed to get professional help.

First Aid Supplies Checklist

Wound Care and Cleaning

Sterile Gauze Pads

Self Adhesive Bandages
i.e., Vetwrap

Wound Cleaners
i.e., Povidone Iodine/ Betadine/ Chlorhexidine/ Saline

Cotton Balls
~Used to help clean wounds

Saline Solution

Medications and Monitoring

Medications
~ Medications prescribed for your pet
~ Triple antibiotic ointment or topical wound spray

Thermometer
Rectal is best - if you are comfortable taking rectal temperatures

Cold Pack/ Hot Pack

E-Collar (Cone)
~Vital for any time we need to keep the cat from licking their body or scratching their head

Safety and Emergency Preparedness

First Aid Tools

Tweezers
~For removing splinters/ stingers/ticks

Disposable gloves

Safety Items

Secure cat carrier

Towel or small blanket
~For restraint, warmth, and calming

Flashlight with extra batteries
~In case you need to locate your pet in the dark

Collapsible Water bowl

Emergency Information

List of medications your cat takes
~Concentration, dosage, frequency

Veterinarian Contact Information

Nearby Emergency Veterinary Facilities

Poison Control Phone #

Figure 1.1. First Aid Supply Checklist

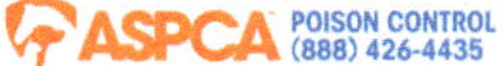

Let's dive a little deeper into some of the items suggested for your first aid kit.

- **Sterile Gauze Pads:**
  - Sterile gauze pads can be applied to wounds to help control bleeding and protect the area from contamination until veterinary care is available.

- **Self-Adhesive Bandages (Vetwrap):**
  - This stretchy bandage sticks to itself and can be useful for securing gauze pads in place or providing light support to an injury.
  - **Important:**
    - With cats, self-adhesive bandages should be used only temporarily and with caution. If applied too tightly or left on too long, they can restrict circulation and worsen injury. Bandages should be removed or replaced promptly once veterinary care is reached.

- **Wound Cleaners:**
  - Povidone Iodine, Betadine, or Chlorhexidine can be used to clean a wound. They will need to be **diluted** prior to use.
    - Wound cleaners may be found in most human pharmacies or purchased online.
    - Apply first to a cotton ball or gauze to clean the area.
  - NEVER use alcohol to flush a wound!
  - AVOID using hydrogen peroxide to clean the wound if at all possible. It stings and can actually delay wound healing.
  - DO NOT attempt to clean wounds that are very deep. In those cases, control bleeding and head to an emergency facility immediately.

Know Your Local ER Options

Emergencies often occur at the worst times and your regular vet might not be available. Knowing the location and contact information of your nearest 24/7 emergency veterinary clinic is crucial to saving time and potentially saving your cat's life.

Locate Your Nearest Emergency Facility

If you are in an area with multiple ERs, locate the two that are closest to you. Ideally, ensure that at least one of the facilities you've written down is open 24/7.

Facility #1	Phone number	Address
__________	__________	__________
__________	__________	__________
Facility #2	Phone number	Address
__________	__________	__________
__________	__________	__________

Map It Out

Know the route to the emergency facility. If possible, drive by the location at least once to become familiar.

Save It

Save the address in your cellphone, along with your regular vet's information. You can even save the address in your GPS!

Have an Emergency Plan

Being prepared for an emergency means having a plan in place before an emergency happens. While not every situation can be anticipated, the following steps can help you respond quickly and effectively:

- **Establish a Plan for Transporting Your Cat:**
  - If your cat is injured or in distress, have a safe method of transport ready. Keep a secure cat carrier easily accessible, along with a towel or blanket to help keep your cat calm and contained during transport.
- **Create a List of Important Contacts:**
  - Keep the following information readily available:
    - Your regular veterinarian
    - The nearest emergency clinic
    - ASPCA Poison Control (888-426-4435)
  - If you're traveling, it's a good idea to research emergency vet clinics along your route and keep their contact details in your car or phone.
- **Make Your Cat's Medical History Accessible:**
  - Keep your cat's medical information easily accessible in case of an emergency. This should include known medical conditions, medications, allergies, emergency instructions, and proof of rabies vaccination. Store this information in your emergency kit, on your phone, or in a digital file, and update it at least once a year.
- **Prepare for Travel with Your Pet:**
  - When traveling with your cat, bring a portable emergency kit with travel-specific items such as extra water, a collapsible bowl, medications, and any supplies your cat may need. Know the location of emergency veterinary clinics along your route and at your destination.

Preparing Your Cat for Care in Your Absence

Traveling can be stressful, especially when leaving your beloved pet in someone else's care. Sadly, emergencies can and do happen when pet owners are traveling. To ensure that your cat receives the fastest and best care while you are away, it's crucial to prepare a comprehensive document with essential information.

Key Information to Include:

1. **Basic Information**
   - Cat's name, age, and breed (especially if exotic)
   - Owner contact information
   - Special care instructions (diet, exercise routine, etc.)
2. **Medications and Health**
   - A list of all medications your pet is currently taking, including dosages and administration times
   - Any known allergies or health conditions (e.g., food allergies, sensitivities)
3. **Veterinary Contacts**
   - Name and contact information for your regular veterinarian
   - Address and phone number of a preferred emergency veterinary facility in case immediate care is needed
4. **Emergency Contact Information**
   - The best phone numbers to reach you
5. **Medical Decision-Making Authorization**
   - Specify whether the caregiver has the authority to make medical decisions on your behalf in case of an emergency. **This authorization can prevent delays in care.**

*A Pet Care & Medical Authorization Form is provided on the following page.

PET CARE & MEDICAL AUTHORIZATION FORM

CAT'S NAME: _______________________

Breed: _______________

Age: _______________

Sex: _______________

Medical Conditions, Allergies:
____

Medications (name/ dosage):
____

Cat Owner Information:

Name: _______________________

Address: _______________________

Phone number(s): _______________________

____

Caregiver Information:

Name: _______________________

Address: _______________________

Phone number(s): _______________________

____

Local Veterinarian Information:

Business Name: _______________________

Address: _______________________

____

Phone #: _______________________

Additional Information: _______________________

____

Preferred Emergency Facility:

Business Name: _______________________

Address: _______________________

____

Phone #: _______________________

Additional Information: _______________________

____

Medical Decision Making Authorization:

☐ I authorize _________________[Caregiver's Name] to make medical decisions for my pet in case of an emergency if I cannot be reached.

☐ I do not authorize _________________[Caregiver's Name] to make medical decisions for my pet in case of an emergency if I cannot be reached.

Completed by: _______________________ Date: _______________

Figure 1.2

Prepare Key Information to Share with the Vet

When contacting your veterinarian or an emergency clinic, they will need specific information to assess the situation and guide next steps. Being prepared with this information can help them provide faster and more effective care. Consider having the following details ready:

Your Pet's Identification Information

- Your cat's name, age, breed
- Any pre-existing medical conditions, current medications, or allergies that might be relevant.

Signs and Timeline

- Describe your cat's signs as clearly and specifically as possible (e.g., "vomiting once every two hours," or "limping after jumping off the couch").
- Provide a timeline for when the signs began or when the incident occurred (such as an injury or toxin exposure).
- Share the information in a logical order, as if you were telling the story of what happened.

Any Interventions Attempted

- Inform the veterinarian of anything you've already tried.

Potential Causes or Exposures

- Share any relevant details, such as possible ingestion, trauma, or exposure to sick animals.

Behavioral Changes or Concerns

- Remember, cats may behave differently at the veterinary clinic. Report any unusual or concerning behaviors you've observed at home.
- Also, no one knows your cat like you do! If something seems concerning/abnormal to you, we want to know!

Figure 1.3: Information to gather for your veterinarian when your cat is sick

SICK VISIT INFO

CAT'S NAME: _______________________

BREED: _________ **AGE:** _____ **MALE/ FEMALE** **INTACT/ ALTERED**

EXISTING MEDICAL CONDITIONS:

____

____

____

____

CURRENT MEDICATIONS:

____

____

____

____

SYMPTOMS:

Include when signs started

____

____

____

____

ANY KNOWN/ SUSPECTED CAUSES:

____

____

____

____

TREATMENTS ALREADY ATTEMPTED:

____

____

____

OTHER CONCERNS:

____

____

____

Printable versions of this chart are available at crittercarecollective.com

A Note About CPR

During an emergency visit, you may be asked about your wishes regarding <u>CPR (Cardiopulmonary Resuscitation)</u> or a DNR (<u>Do Not Resuscitate</u>) order. This is a **routine question** in emergency settings and is often asked as part of standard emergency intake, regardless of how stable a cat may appear.

This question can feel stressful, but it is asked so the veterinary team understands your wishes if an unexpected emergency occurs. Because conditions can change quickly, CPR preferences are often discussed early, sometimes before you speak directly with the veterinarian.

What Does CPR Look Like?

In the unlikely and unfortunate situation where a cat experiences cardiac or respiratory arrest and CPR has been elected, the veterinary team will begin immediate resuscitation efforts with the goal of restoring breathing and circulation.

CPR may include:
- Chest compressions to attempt to circulate blood
- Placement of a breathing tube and assisted ventilation
- Administration of emergency medications to attempt to support heart function

*CPR is an invasive emergency procedure and may cause physical injury, such as rib fractures, which would need to be managed if the cat survives.

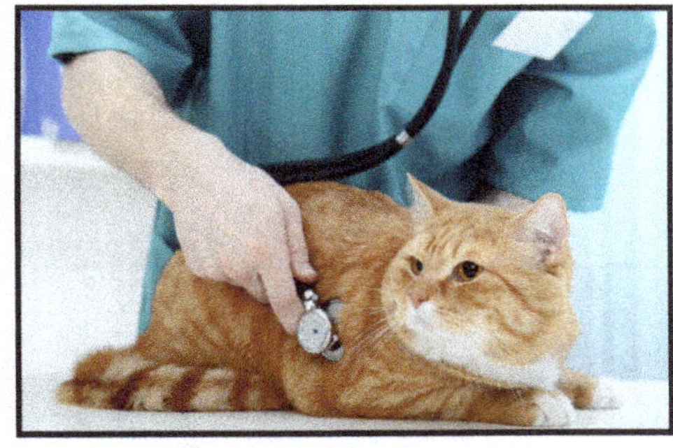

A Note About CPR Outcomes

Cardiac or respiratory arrest is always caused by a serious underlying problem. Outcomes after CPR depend on factors such as:

- the severity of the underlying illness or injury
- the length of time circulation or oxygen delivery was impaired
- existing medical conditions
- whether the cause of arrest can be reversed

CPR in cats has a low success rate when measured by how many cats survive long enough to leave the hospital. Even with rapid intervention and skilled care, the likelihood of a cat surviving cardiac arrest and returning home is limited. Better outcomes are more often seen in rare situations, such as arrest during anesthesia or when the cause can be quickly reversed.

Making the Decision

There is no right or wrong choice when it comes to CPR. Some families elect CPR, while others choose a comfort-based approach and select DNR. This decision is personal.

While emergencies cannot be predicted, having a basic understanding of what CPR involves and considering how you would prefer to proceed if cardiac or respiratory arrest were to occur can help guide decisions if the situation arises unexpectedly.

Veterinary teams will always focus on stabilizing your cat and preventing emergencies whenever possible.

A Practical Consideration

It is also important to be aware that CPR and subsequent critical care involve significant medical resources and may carry a substantial financial cost, particularly if ongoing hospitalization is required after resuscitation.

Pet Insurance Benefits

As a devoted cat owner, you want the best for your cat. Unexpected veterinary costs can add up quickly, especially during emergencies. Pet insurance can serve as a valuable financial safety net, offering peace of mind and helping manage the cost of veterinary care. Benefits include:

- Financial Protection Against High Costs
    - Emergency care for cats can be expensive. Pet insurance may cover a significant portion of these costs, making urgent care more accessible.
- Access to Quality Care
    - With pet insurance, medical decisions can be based on your cat's health needs rather than financial limitations. This can reduce delays in care and improve outcomes.
- Preventive Care Options
    - Some pet insurance plans offer coverage for preventive care, such as routine exams, vaccinations, and dental cleanings, which can help maintain long-term health and reduce the risk of costly illness.

Enroll When Your Cat is Young and Healthy

The best time to enroll in pet insurance is when your cat is young. Premiums are typically lower and coverage is more comprehensive since pre-existing conditions are less likely.

It's important to note that most pet insurance policies do not cover pre-existing conditions. If your cat is diagnosed with an illness before enrollment, related treatments are usually excluded from coverage.

Many pet insurance companies are available. Talk with your veterinarian about your cat's needs and which insurance options may be a good fit.

TEN MOST COMMON EMERGENCIES

Emergencies can happen without warning, and knowing how to respond is an important part of caring for your cat. In this chapter, we'll focus on the ten most common emergencies seen in cats, ranging from frequently encountered problems to life-threatening conditions. You'll learn how to recognize early warning signs, understand potential causes, and know when immediate veterinary care is needed.

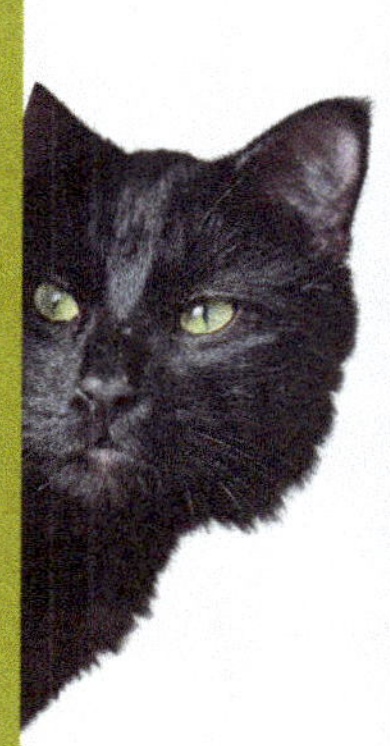

Chapter Highlights

Top 10 Emergencies:

1. Abscess
2. Linear Foreign Body
3. Congestive Heart Failure
4. Urinary Obstruction
5. Kidney Failure
6. Diabetic Ketoacidosis (DKA)
7. Constipation
8. Upper Respiratory Infection (URI)
9. Severe Anemia
10. Trauma

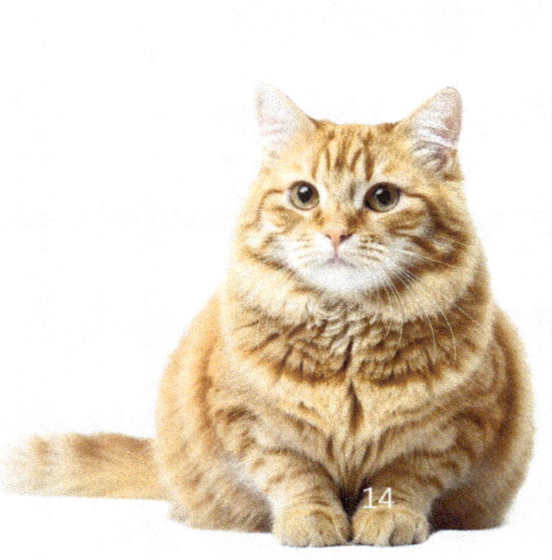

ABSCESS

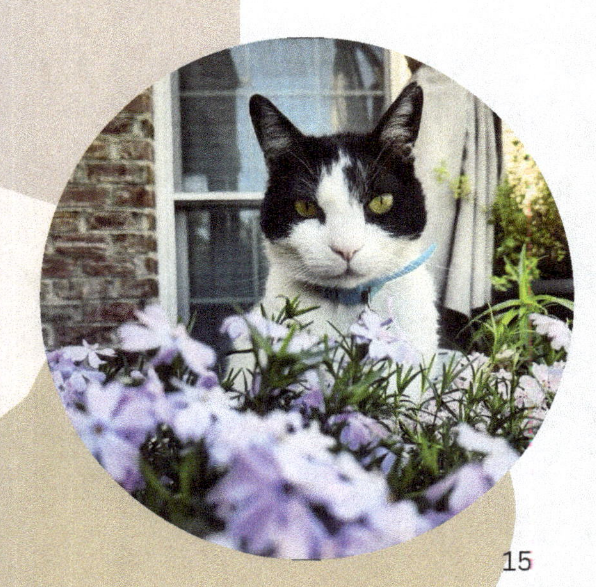

What's an Abscess?

An abscess is a pocket of pus that forms when bacteria enter the body through a break in the skin—most often due to a bite or puncture wound. In cats, especially those allowed outdoors, abscesses typically result from cat fights. As the body reacts to the infection, pus accumulates under the skin, creating a swollen, painful area. Over time, the abscess may rupture and drain or cause more widespread infection.

Cats Most Affected

Any cat may develop an abscess. However, those most predisposed include:

- Cats who spend time outdoors
- Intact male cats
- Territorial male cats
- Cats in high-density homes or feral colonies

Signs of an Abscess

Recognizing the signs of an abscess can help you seek care before the infection worsens. Common signs include:

- **Localized, rapidly growing swelling**
  - This can be anywhere on the body; however, they are very often on the face, tail base, or limbs.
- **Warmth or pain when touched**
- **Oozing pus or blood**
  - Many abscesses are first noticed after they rupture and begin to drain.
- **Licking or chewing at the affected area**
- **Fever, lethargy, or decreased appetite**
- **Hiding**
- **Limping**
  - This is seen if the abscess is located on a leg.

If you suspect your cat has an abscess, please do the following:

- Keep your cat indoors and away from other animals.
- Do not attempt to lance or drain the abscess yourself.
- Contact your veterinarian to schedule an immediate visit.
  - If your regular veterinarian is unable to see your cat promptly, seek care at an urgent care clinic or emergency hospital.
- Transport your cat in a secure carrier to prevent injury and reduce stress.

Common Interventions:

At the veterinary clinic/hospital, you may expect the following:

- **Veterinary Examination:** A thorough physical exam will be performed, along with discussion of your cat's history.
- **Sedation or Anesthesia:** Light sedation or anesthesia may be required to safely clip the fur, and to clean and flush the area.
- **Lancing and Drainage:** If an abscess is present, it is typically opened, drained, and flushed to remove infected material.
- **Medications:** Oral or injectable antibiotics are commonly prescribed, along with pain medications and anti-inflammatories to manage discomfort and infection.
- **Protective Measures:** An Elizabethan collar (e-collar) may be recommended for several days to prevent licking or trauma while the wound heals.
- **Home Care Instructions:** You may be given guidance for home care, such as applying warm compresses, keeping the area clean, and monitoring the wound. Cats are often advised to remain indoors during the healing period.

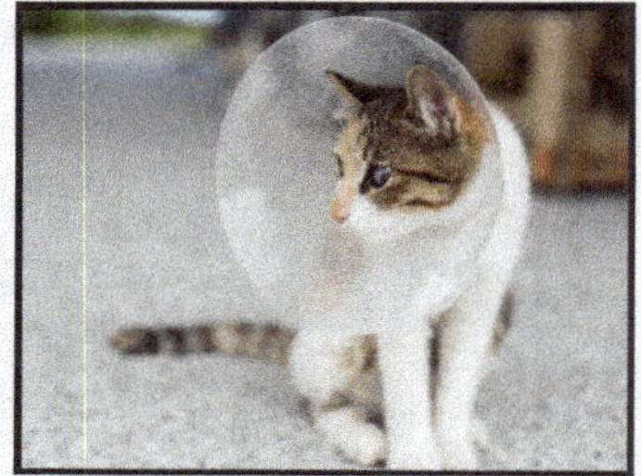

Prevention

Abscesses are not always preventable; however, the following steps may help reduce risk:

- **Keep cats indoors.** Indoor cats are less likely to be involved in fights that result in bite wounds.
    - **Outdoor access considerations:** If you choose to allow your cat outdoors, ensure they are spayed or neutered and kept up to date on recommended vaccinations.
- **Spay or neuter cats.** This can reduce roaming and territorial aggression, lowering the risk of injuries.
- **Manage multi-cat households.** If cats are prone to fighting, ensure each cat has access to their own space, hiding areas, and resources. Environmental enrichment and stimulation can help reduce tension. Veterinary or behavioral guidance may be helpful if aggression persists. Separation may be considered in severe cases.
- **Seek veterinary care promptly for suspected wounds.** If a bite or injury is suspected, it is best to see a veterinarian sooner rather than waiting.
    - Wounds, especially bite wounds, often become infected quickly, even if they appear minor at first.

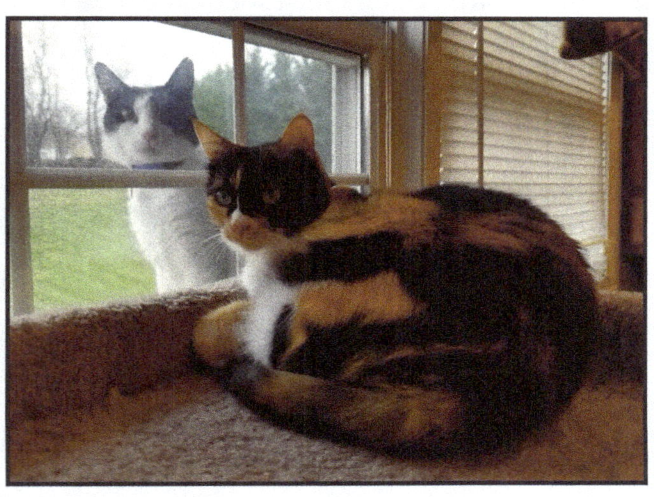

LINEAR FOREIGN BODY

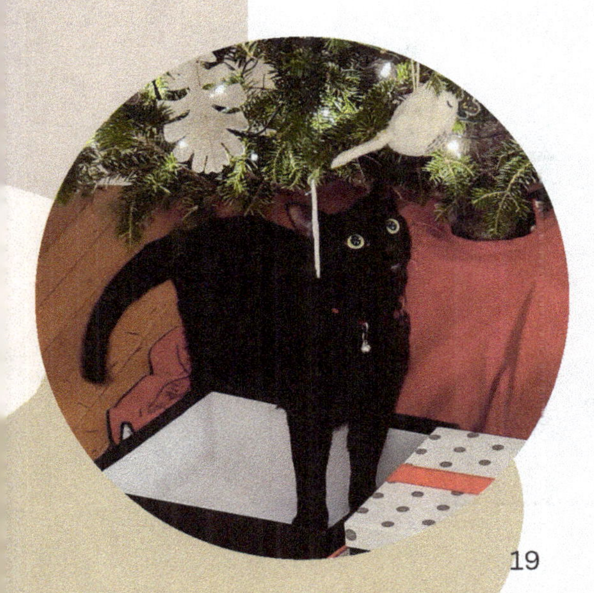

True Emergency

What is a Linear Foreign Body?

Vomiting is a common reason cats are brought to the veterinarian and can have many causes, ranging from mild issues to life-threatening conditions. One particularly serious cause is ingestion of a linear foreign body, such as string, thread, yarn, or tinsel, which requires immediate veterinary attention.

A linear foreign body is a long, string-like object that becomes trapped in the gastrointestinal tract. In cats, these objects often become caught under the tongue or in the stomach while the other end continues to move through the intestines. This causes the intestines to "accordion," which can lead to tearing, perforation, or rupture.

Because cats are naturally inclined to chew on string-like objects, they are especially vulnerable to this emergency.

Cats Most Affected

- Curious kittens and young cats
- Cats with access to sewing supplies, gift wrap, or string-based toys
- Cats prone to eating non-food items (pica)

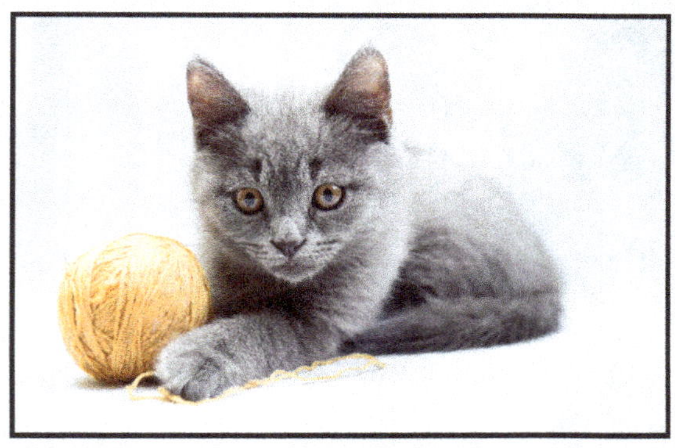

Signs of a Linear Foreign Body

Knowing the signs of a linear foreign body emergency is critical, as early recognition can help prevent serious complications. Clinical signs can vary, and not all cats will show every sign listed below:

- **Repeated vomiting,** often without food or only fluid
- **Painful or tense abdomen**
- **Hiding, lethargy, or weakness**
- **Anorexia** with decreased or absent appetite
- **String visible under the tongue or protruding from the anus**
  - This is an emergency. *DO NOT attempt to pull on the string.*
- **Pawing at the mouth or drooling**
- **Known or suspected ingestion** of string, thread, or similar objects (even if signs are mild)

What Can You Do?

If your cat is vomiting, hiding, showing abdominal discomfort, or you suspect ingestion of a string or similar object, please do the following:

- **Do not** pull on any visible string from the mouth or anus, as this can cause severe internal injury.
- Keep your cat calm and limit movement and handling.
- **Seek emergency veterinary care immediately.**

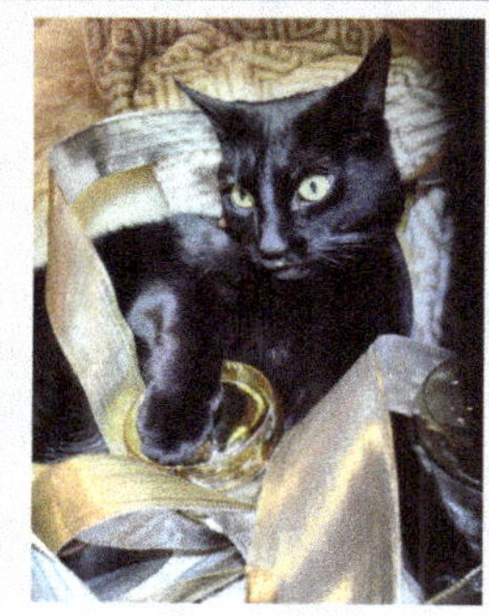

Ribbons, tinsel, and string can be extremely dangerous for cats and may cause a serious medical emergency if swallowed.

At the veterinary clinic or hospital, you may expect the following:

- **Veterinary Examination:** A thorough physical exam will be performed, along with discussion of your cat's history and recent signs.
- **Sedation or Anesthesia:** May be required to safely examine the mouth (including under the tongue) and to perform diagnostic imaging.
- **Diagnostic Imaging:** X-rays and/or ultrasound services are commonly used to identify the foreign body and assess intestinal involvement.
- **Emergency Surgery:** Surgery is frequently required to remove the linear foreign body.
  - Unlike some other surgical conditions, linear foreign bodies pose an imminent risk of intestinal damage or perforation and are therefore typically treated as a surgical emergency.
- **Supportive Care:** IV fluids, antibiotics, and pain medications are commonly administered.

Prevention

Linear foreign bodies are not always preventable, as cats are curious and often ingest items without being seen. However, the following steps may help reduce risk:

- **Store string-like items out of reach.** This includes thread, yarn, floss, rubber bands, ribbon, and hair ties.
- **Discard damaged toys promptly.** Remove loose strings or frayed parts.
- **Supervise play with wand toys** and put them away after use.
- **Avoid tinsel** and similar decorations, especially during holidays.

CONGESTIVE HEART FAILURE

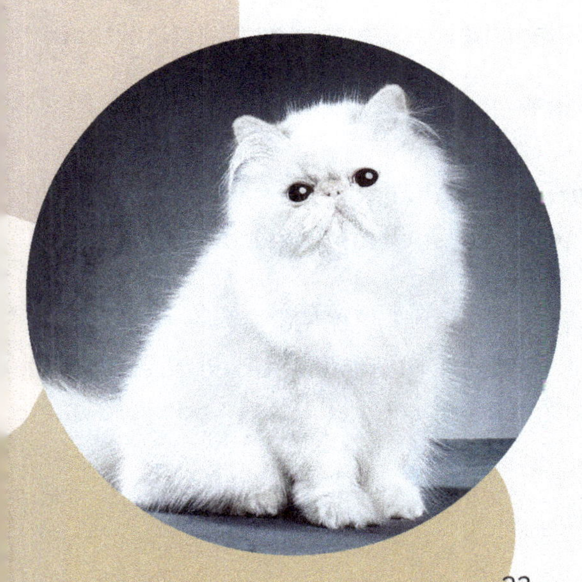

True Emergency

What is Congestive Heart Failure (CHF)?

Congestive heart failure (CHF) occurs when the heart can no longer pump blood effectively, leading to fluid buildup in or around the lungs. In cats, the most common underlying cause is hypertrophic cardiomyopathy (HCM), a condition in which the heart muscle becomes abnormally thickened and stiff, interfering with normal filling and breathing.

Cats Most Affected

Congestive heart failure can occur in any cat; however, certain breeds are more commonly affected due to a higher prevalence of hypertrophic cardiomyopathy (HCM), the most common underlying cause of CHF in cats.

Breeds with increased risk include:

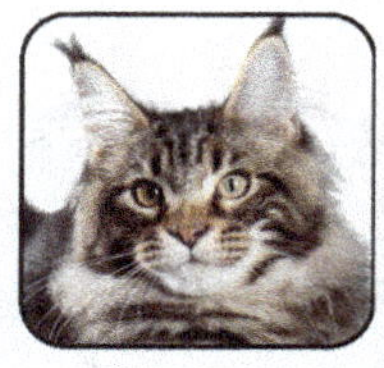

Maine Coon

Ragdoll

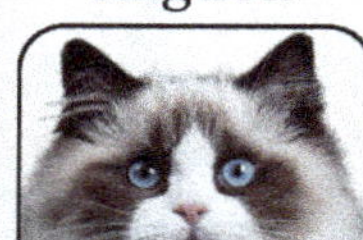

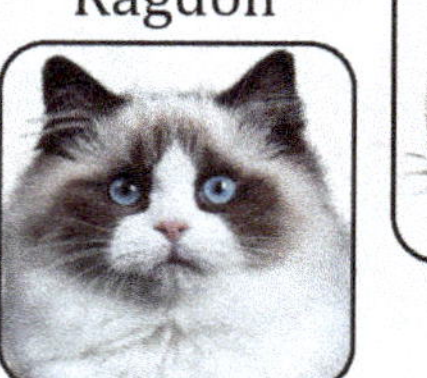

British Shorthair

Sphynx

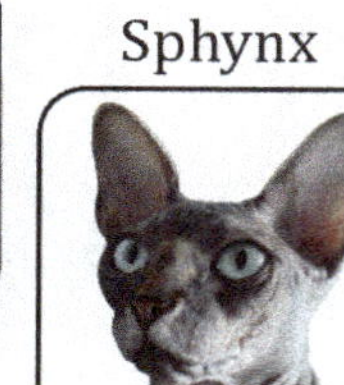

American Shorthair

Additional cats at increased risk include:
- Middle-aged to older cats
- Cats with known heart murmurs or diagnosed heart disease
- Cats with underlying conditions, such as hyperthyroidism or high blood pressure

While certain breeds are more commonly affected, mixed-breed cats can also develop HCM, and absence of breed risk does not rule out congestive heart failure.

<h1 align="center">Signs of CHF</h1>

Knowing the signs of congestive heart failure is critical, as this condition can rapidly become life-threatening. Clinical signs can vary, and not all cats will show every sign listed below:

- **Increased breathing rate or effort:** Rapid, shallow, or labored breathing
- **Open-mouth breathing or panting:** Always abnormal in cats
- **Lethargy or weakness**
- **Decreased appetite**
- **Hiding or reduced activity**
- **Collapse or sudden weakness**
- **Pale or bluish gums:** A sign of poor oxygenation

<h1 align="center">Common Causes of CHF</h1>

There are several conditions that can lead to congestive heart failure in cats. Common causes include:

- **Hypertrophic Cardiomyopathy (HCM):**
  - This is the most common cause of CHF in cats. The heart muscle becomes thickened and stiff, impairing normal filling and leading to fluid buildup.
- **Other Cardiomyopathies:**
  - Less commonly, cats may develop dilated, restrictive, or unclassified cardiomyopathies that impair heart function.
- **Congenital Heart Defects:**
  - Some cats are born with structural heart abnormalities that may eventually lead to CHF
- **Secondary Heart Disease:**
  - Conditions such as hyperthyroidism or systemic hypertension (high blood pressure) can place added strain on the heart and contribute to heart failure.

Signs of congestive heart failure involve respiratory distress, which is a true emergency and requires immediate care.

- **Contact a veterinarian immediately:** Call your veterinarian or an emergency clinic to let them know you are on your way. Confirm that the facility can provide oxygen support and hospitalization.
- **Keep your cat calm:** Minimize stress and handling while preparing for transport.
- **Avoid activity:** Keep your cat quiet and confined. Do not encourage movement or play, as exertion can worsen breathing difficulty.

Common Interventions:

At the veterinary hospital, the following treatments may be provided:

- **Oxygen Therapy:** This is often required to stabilize breathing.
- **Medications:** They are commonly used during initial stabilization and may include:
  - Anti-anxiety or mild sedation to reduce stress and breathing effort
  - Diuretics to reduce fluid buildup in or around the lungs
  - Additional heart medications to support heart function or manage blood pressure
- **Diagnostic Testing:** Chest X-rays are typically performed to assess fluid accumulation, and blood work may be recommended to evaluate overall stability.
- **Cardiology Referral:** Once stabilized, referral for an echocardiogram (heart ultrasound) may be recommended to confirm the underlying heart disease and guide long-term care.

Congestive heart failure is not always preventable, particularly when caused by underlying heart disease. However, early detection and management may help reduce the risk of severe complications.

- **Routine veterinary exams:** They may identify heart murmurs or early changes before clinical signs develop.
- **Management of underlying conditions:** They may include hyperthyroidism or high blood pressure.
- **Early heart screening:** Proactive heart evaluation is recommended in breeds with higher risk for HCM.
- **Prompt evaluation of breathing changes:** Early intervention may improve outcomes.

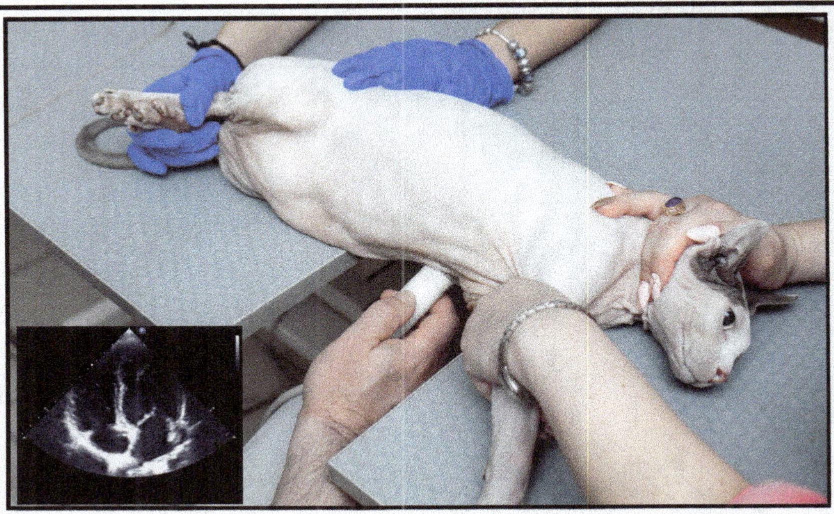

Figure 2.1. Evaluation by a cardiologist using an echocardiogram (ultrasound of the heart) is very helpful for cats with heart disease. Ideally, this is performed when heart disease is first suspected or identified. Follow-up evaluation after diagnosis is important to guide medication decisions.

Cats experiencing breathing difficulty often require immediate oxygen support and may be taken directly to the treatment area upon arrival.

There are several methods for providing oxygen. In some cases, oxygen is delivered temporarily using a mask or flow-by oxygen held near the face (see Figures 2.2 and 2.3). This is typically a short-term measure that allows the veterinary team to begin stabilization while obtaining critical information, placing an intravenous catheter, collecting blood samples, or performing diagnostic tests.

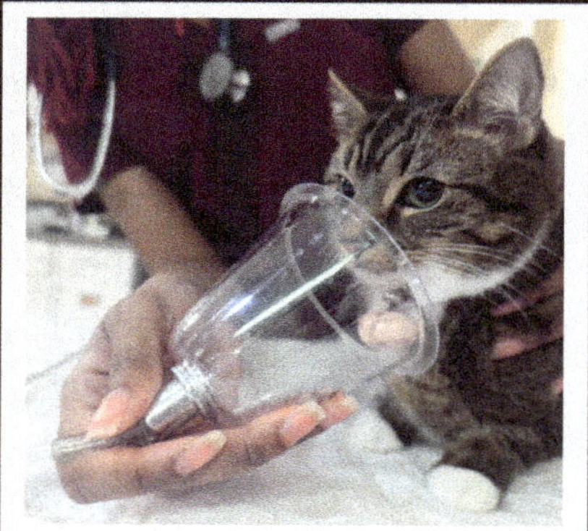

Figure 2.2. Cat receiving O2 via face mask

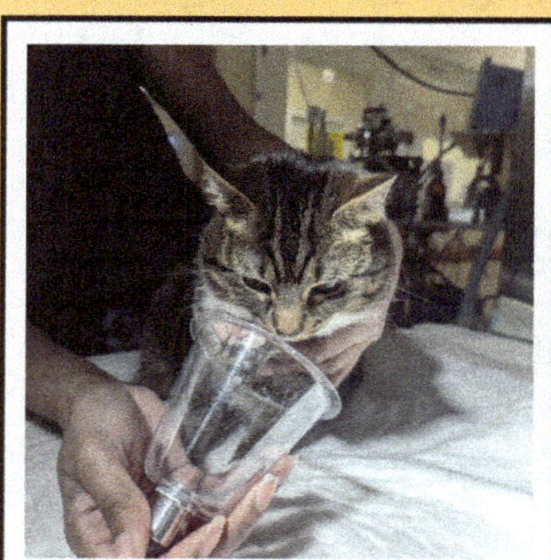

Figure 2.3. Cat receiving oxygen via mask/ flow-by

Most cats with respiratory distress will not be able to go home right away. It often takes time to stabilize breathing and address the underlying cause. Because cats generally do not tolerate masks or restraint well, they are commonly transitioned to an oxygen kennel once immediate hands-on care is complete.

Oxygen kennels offer several advantages for cats. They allow oxygen supplementation without restraint or repeated handling, which is especially important for reducing stress. Temperature and humidity can be carefully controlled, and the enclosed, quiet environment helps block out the noise and activity of a busy emergency clinic. Many cats breathe more comfortably once settled in this calm setting (Fig 2.4).

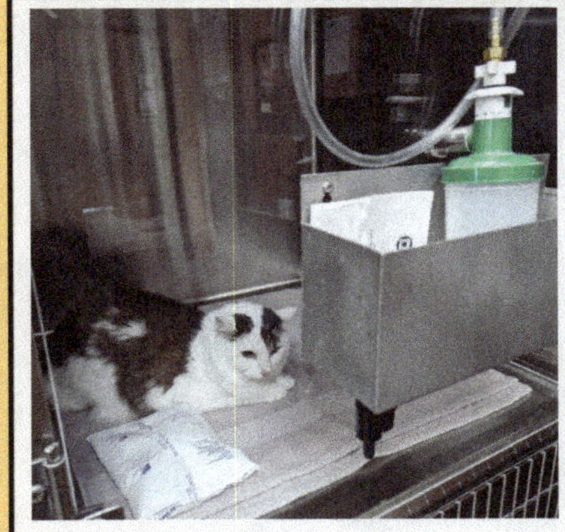

Figure 2.4. Cat in O2 cage. Administration of oxygen via oxygen cages is often well tolerated in cats.

Photo credit: Dr. B. Castillo; "Panda"

Note:

There may be times when visitation is discouraged while your cat is receiving oxygen support. For cats in significant respiratory distress, seeing their owner can increase excitement or anxiety, which may worsen breathing. During these critical moments, minimizing stimulation allows your cat to focus on breathing and recovery.

URINARY OBSTRUCTION

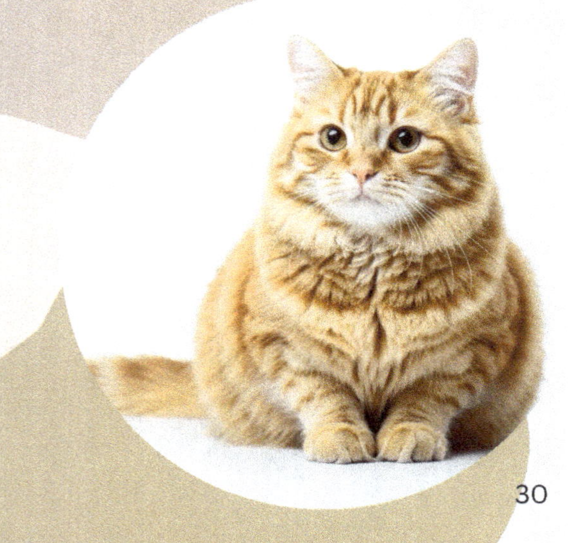

What is a Urinary Obstruction?

A urinary obstruction occurs when a cat is unable to pass urine due to a blockage in the urethra, the tube that carries urine out of the bladder. This condition is most common in male cats, whose urethra is narrower and more easily obstructed.

Blockages are typically caused by a combination of mucus, urinary crystals, small stones, or inflammation associated with **Feline Idiopathic Cystitis (FIC)**. As urine backs up in the bladder, toxins accumulate in the bloodstream and electrolyte levels become dangerously abnormal.

If not treated promptly, urinary obstruction can lead to kidney failure, life-threatening heart rhythm abnormalities, collapse, or death. **Urinary obstruction is one of the most urgent emergencies in feline medicine.**

Cats Most Affected

While any cat can become obstructed, certain cats are at higher risk:

- **Male cats,** especially neutered males
- **Young to middle-aged cats,** typically 2–7 years old
- **Indoor-only cats** with limited activity
- **Cats with a history of FIC**
  - **Cats with low water intake,** especially those only on a dry-food diet
- **Cats in multi-cat households or high-stress environments**
- **Overweight or obese cats**

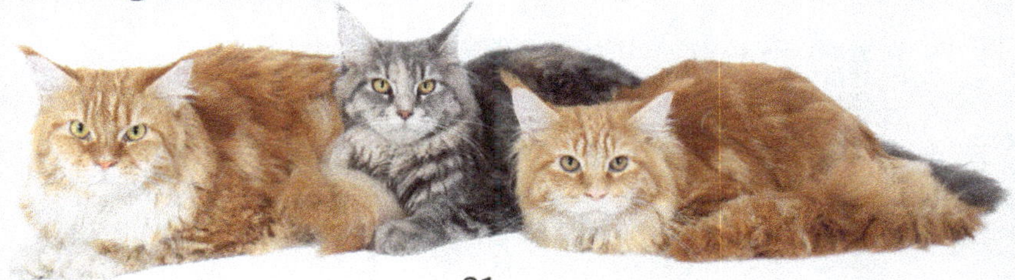

Urinary obstruction is often mistaken for constipation. Early recognition is critical.

- **Straining in the litter box** with little or no urine produced
- **Frequent trips to the litter box**
- **Crying or vocalizing** while attempting to urinate
    - Cats are often described as "yowling" when they have this condition.
- **Lethargy or hiding**
- **Vomiting**
- **Excessive licking of the genital area**
- **Firm or distended abdomen**
    - This finding can be subtle and is not always noticeable to owners, especially early in the course of obstruction
- **Collapse or sudden weakness** if the obstruction has been present too long

If you suspect urinary concerns in your cat, especially a **male cat:**

- **Contact your veterinarian** immediately to discuss the signs and determine next steps.
    - If your veterinarian is unavailable, proceed to an **emergency facility.**
- **Minimize stress and handling.** Transport your cat in a secure carrier and avoid pressure on the abdomen.
- **Know what is normal for your cat.**
    - Learning how to gently palpate your cat's bladder ahead of time can help you recognize when something isn't right.
        - See your Emergency Toolkit section for a refresher (page 114).

Common Interventions:

At the veterinary clinic or hospital, you may expect the following:

- **Veterinary Examination:** A thorough physical exam will be performed. The diagnosis can often be made by identifying a large, firm bladder that cannot be emptied with gentle pressure.

- **IV Catheter Placement and Initial Stabilization:** An IV catheter will typically be placed early with blood work obtained to assess kidney function and electrolytes. If severe abnormalities or heart rhythm changes are detected, stabilization will be prioritized.

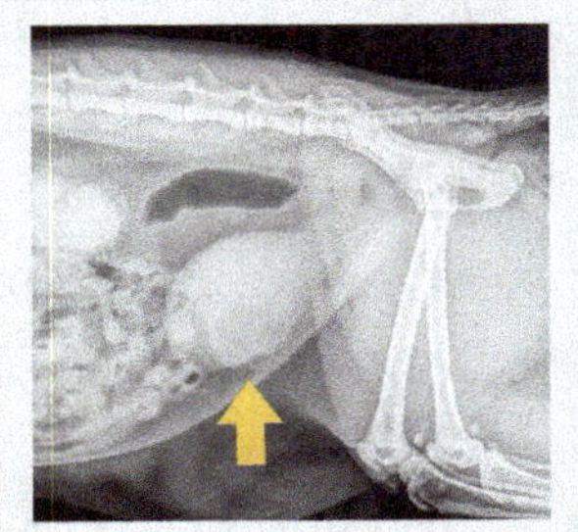

Figure 2.5. X-ray showing a typical cat urinary bladder

- **Sedation and Urinary Catheterization:** Sedation or anesthesia is typically required to place a urinary catheter, relieve the obstruction, and empty the bladder.

- **Bladder and Urethral Flushing:** The bladder and urethra will be flushed to remove mucus, crystals, debris, or small stones.

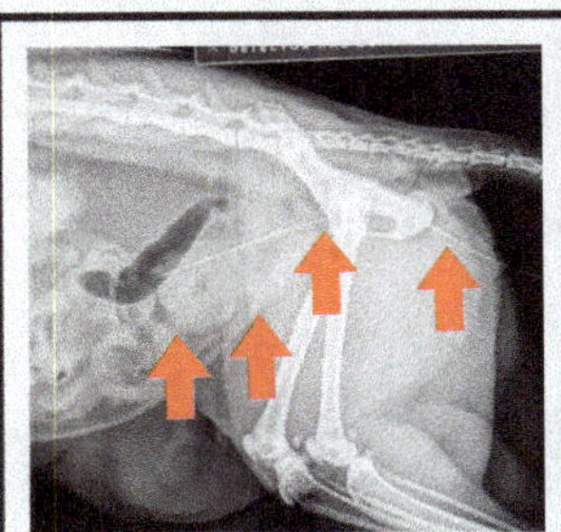

Figure 2.6. X-ray showing a urinary catheter inserted into a cat bladder

- **Additional Testing:** Additional testing is often performed, including more complete blood work, urinalysis, and radiographs (X-rays) to evaluate for bladder or urethral stones and to confirm appropriate urinary catheter placement.

- **Hospitalization:** Ongoing monitoring, IV fluid therapy, and urine output measurement are commonly required for one or more days.

- **Medications:** Pain control and medications to reduce urethral spasm or inflammation are commonly administered.

- **Dietary Recommendations:** Prescription urinary diets may be recommended to reduce the risk of recurrence.

Urinary obstruction cannot always be prevented, but several strategies may reduce risk, particularly in male cats and cats with a history of urinary disease:

- **Adequate hydration:** Encouraging water intake helps dilute urine and reduce crystal and plug formation. This may include feeding canned food, adding water to meals, or providing water fountains.
- **Stress management:** Stress is a known contributor to FIC. Maintaining a predictable routine, providing environmental enrichment, and minimizing household stressors are important preventive measures.
- **Litter box management:** Proper litter box setup plays an important role in urinary health.
    - Litter boxes should be placed in quiet locations away from sudden, loud, or unpredictable noises, such as washing machines, dryers, or high-traffic areas.
    - Some cats have strong preferences for litter box style. Experimenting with open versus covered boxes may be helpful.
    - Automatic or self-cleaning litter boxes work well for some cats but may be stressful for others. Non-electric boxes may be better tolerated in noise-sensitive cats.
    - Providing **one litter box per cat plus one extra** is commonly recommended.
    - Litter boxes should be kept clean and easily accessible at all times.
- **Litter type preferences:** Many cats prefer unscented litter.
- **Healthy body weight and activity:** Maintaining a healthy weight and encouraging regular activity may help reduce risk factors associated with urinary disease.
- **Early recognition of signs:** Prompt veterinary evaluation for straining, frequent litter box visits, or changes in urination may help prevent progression to complete obstruction.

- **Dietary modification:** Prescription urinary diets are commonly recommended after an obstruction to reduce the risk of recurrence, depending on the underlying cause.
- **Ongoing hydration support:** Increasing water intake remains a critical long-term strategy after recovery.
- **Medical management when indicated:** Some cats may require medications to manage inflammation, pain, urethral spasm, or stress-related bladder disease.
- **Close monitoring:** Cats with a history of obstruction are at increased risk for recurrence. Careful observation for early signs allows for faster intervention.

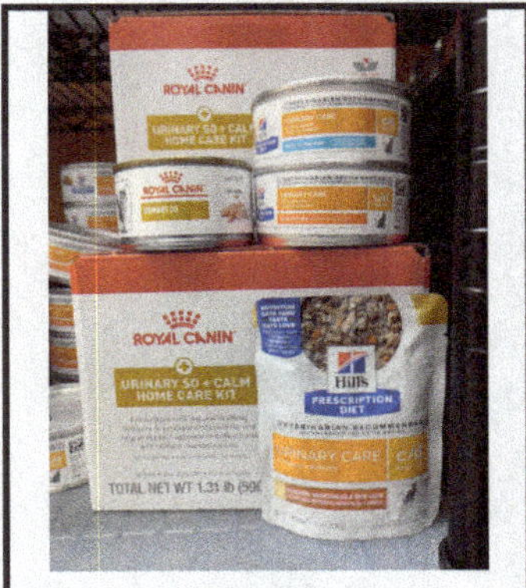

Your veterinarian may recommend a therapeutic urinary diet to help manage and prevent urinary problems.

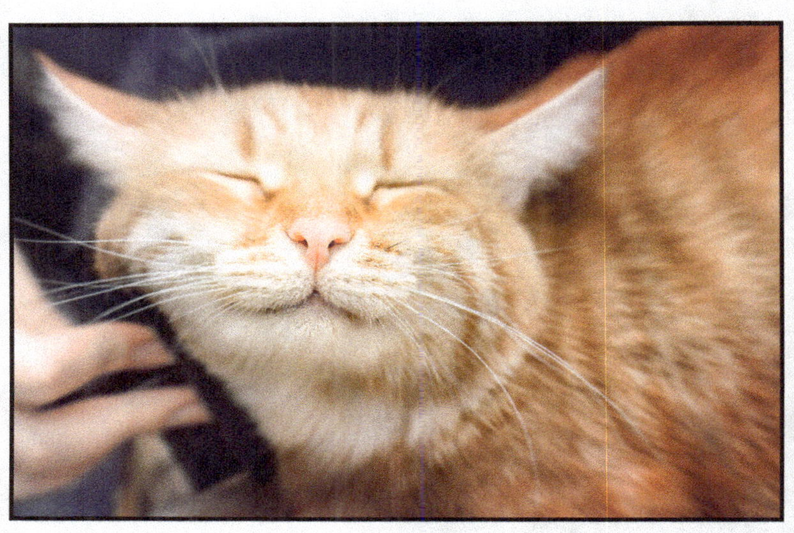

KIDNEY FAILURE

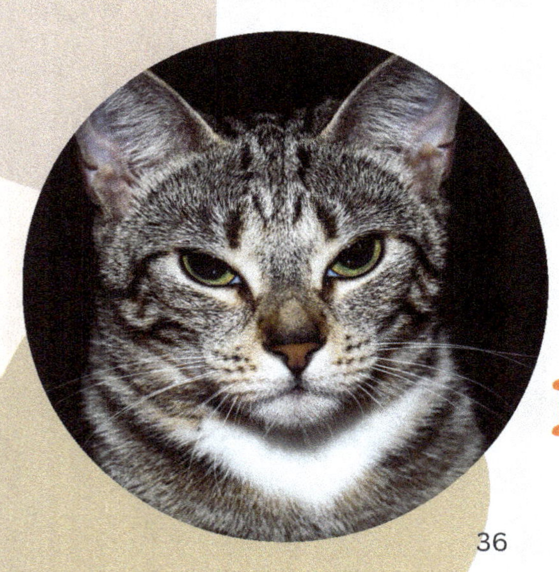

ACUTE KIDNEY INJURY (AKI)

True Emergency

Kidney failure occurs when the kidneys lose their ability to filter waste products, regulate fluids and electrolytes, and maintain normal body balance.

In emergency settings, this most often refers to **acute kidney injury (AKI)**, which develops rapidly over hours to days and can be life-threatening without prompt treatment.

AKI differs from chronic kidney disease, which develops slowly over time. Cats with underlying kidney disease are more vulnerable to sudden worsening and acute decompensation.

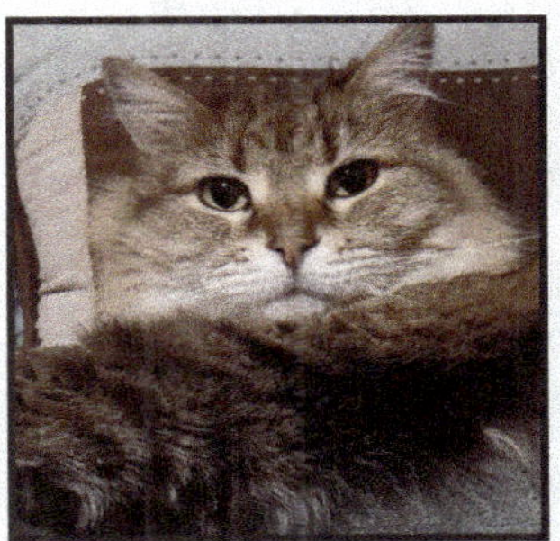

Cats Most Affected

Kidney failure can occur in cats of any age. While it is more common in adult and senior cats, younger cats may also be affected due to congenital or genetic abnormalities, toxin exposure, or severe illness. Certain cats are at higher risk, including:

- Adult and senior cats
- Cats with pre-existing kidney disease
- Cats exposed to toxins (such as certain medications, plants, or chemicals)
- Cats with severe dehydration, shock, or trauma
- Cats with urinary obstruction or severe infection

Signs of Kidney Failure

Signs of kidney failure may develop suddenly or worsen quickly and can vary depending on the underlying cause and severity. You may notice:

- **Decreased appetite or refusal to eat:** Cats with kidney failure are often nauseated and are hence uninterested in food.
- **Vomiting:** Vomiting may occur and can become more frequent as the condition worsens.
- **Lethargy or weakness:** Cats may seem unusually tired, withdrawn, or less active.
- **Increased drinking and urination:** Drinking more water and urinating larger volumes are common early warning signs of kidney disease and should prompt veterinary evaluation.
- **Changes in urination:** As the condition progresses, some cats may urinate less or stop producing urine altogether, which is a more serious sign.
- **Dehydration:** Cats may become dehydrated even if water intake appears normal (see page 133 for dehydration assessment).
- **Weight loss:** Rapid or unexplained weight loss may occur.
- **Drooling or mouth discomfort:** Excessive drooling, bad breath, or mouth sores may be present in more severe cases.

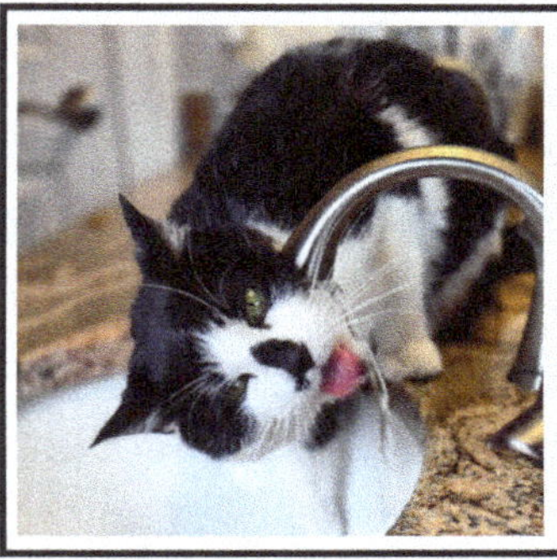

Increased drinking is frequently seen in cats with kidney disease but may also occur with other illnesses, so veterinary evaluation is recommended.

Because the signs of kidney failure can be vague and may overlap with many other conditions, prompt veterinary evaluation is important when changes in drinking, urination, appetite, or behavior are noted.

- **Contact your veterinarian** promptly to discuss the signs and determine next steps.
    - If your veterinarian is unavailable, proceed to an emergency veterinary facility.
- **Minimize stress and handling:** Transport your cat in a secure carrier and keep them warm and calm during travel.
- **Know what is normal**: Being familiar with your cat's normal drinking, urination, appetite, and energy levels can help identify concerning changes earlier.

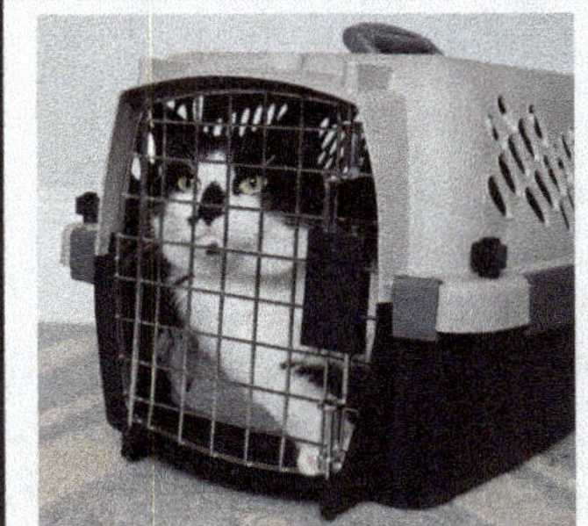

Cats should always be transported in a carrier to keep them safe and secure during veterinary visits.

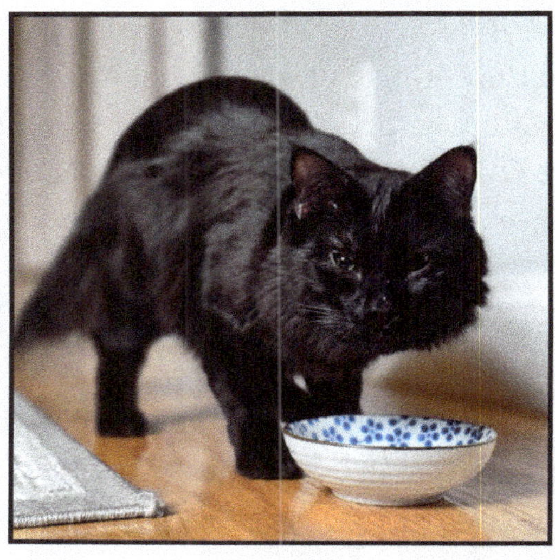

At the veterinary clinic or hospital, you may expect the following:

- **Veterinary Examination:** A thorough physical exam will be performed, along with review of recent changes in drinking, urination, appetite, toxin exposure, and medical history.
- **IV Catheter Placement**: An IV catheter will be placed early to allow for blood sampling, fluid therapy, and supportive care.
- **Blood Work and Urinalysis:** Blood tests and urinalysis are commonly performed to assess kidney function, electrolyte status, hydration, and to help determine severity and possible causes.
- **Fluid Therapy:** IV fluids are a cornerstone of treatment and are used to support circulation, correct dehydration, and help improve kidney function when possible.
- **Diagnostic Imaging:** X-rays and/or ultrasound may be performed to evaluate kidney size and structure and to look for stones or other abnormalities affecting the urinary tract.

Figure 2.7. IV access via catheterization is typically one of the first procedures initiated, as intravenous fluids are a cornerstone of therapy for kidney injury.

- **Hospitalization**: Ongoing monitoring, IV fluid therapy, and repeat laboratory testing are often required for several days.
- **Supportive Care:** Additional supportive treatments may be provided based on the individual cat's needs and response to therapy.

Not all causes of kidney failure can be prevented, but several steps may reduce risk and support kidney health.

- **Ensure adequate hydration:** Encouraging regular water intake helps support kidney function. This may include feeding canned food, adding water to meals, or using water fountains.
- **Be cautious with toxin exposure**: Many substances can damage the kidneys if ingested, even in small amounts.
  - **Familiarize yourself with common toxins:** Knowing which plants, medications, foods, and household products are dangerous to cats can help prevent accidental exposure. See Chapter 3 for a listing of the ten most common toxicities.
- **Use medications carefully**: Only give medications as prescribed by a veterinarian.
  - There are no over-the-counter medications proven to be safe for cats without veterinary guidance.
- **Recognize early warning signs:** Changes in drinking, urination, appetite, energy level, or behavior should prompt veterinary evaluation.
- **Routine veterinary care:** Regular wellness exams and screening blood work, especially in adult and senior cats, may help identify kidney changes earlier.
  - As cats age, yearly or twice-yearly visits are encouraged to help identify kidney changes early.
- **Support cats with existing kidney disease:** In cats with known kidney disease, ongoing veterinary monitoring is especially important. Some cats may benefit from more frequent exams, specialized diets, or medications based on disease progression and individual needs.

DIABETIC KETOACIDOSIS

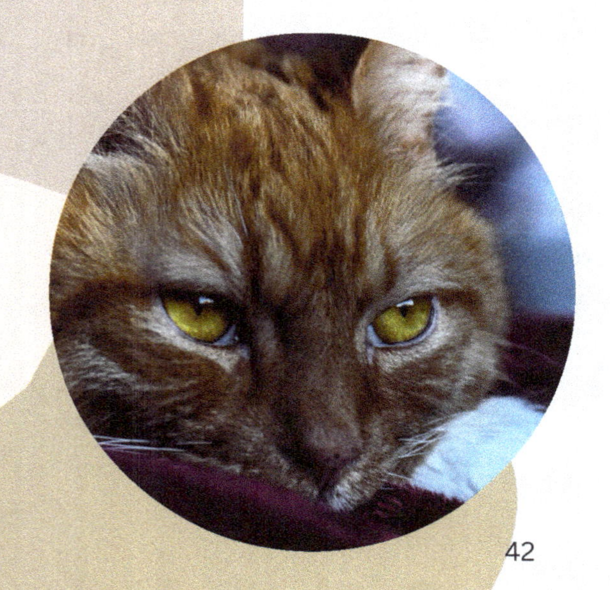

DKA

True Emergency

What is Diabetic Ketoacidosis (DKA)?

Diabetic ketoacidosis occurs when the body lacks enough insulin to use sugar for energy. When this happens, the body begins breaking down fat instead. This process is inefficient and leads to the buildup of ketones, which are byproducts of fat metabolism. As ketones accumulate, they cause serious metabolic disturbances and lead to severe illness.

Cats Most Affected

DKA can occur in any cat with diabetes. While many affected cats have a known diagnosis, some cats develop DKA before diabetes has been formally diagnosed. This may occur for a variety of reasons, including subtle early signs or delayed recognition.
Risk is higher in:

- Cats with newly diagnosed or previously unrecognized diabetes
- Cats that have missed insulin doses
- Cats with diabetes that is not yet well regulated
- Cats with concurrent illness, such as infection, pancreatitis, kidney disease, or liver disease

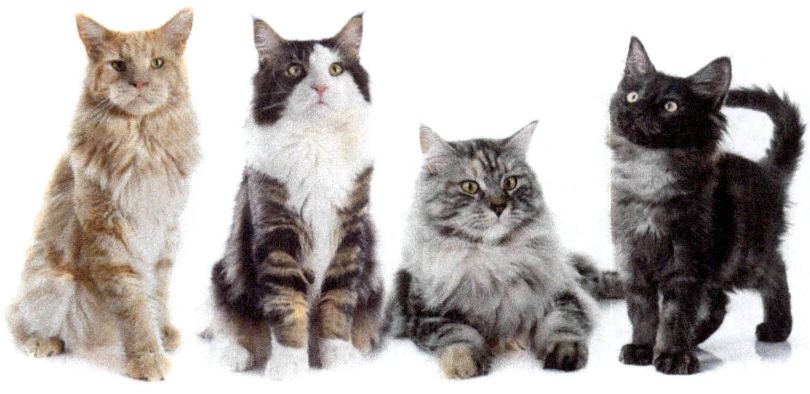

Signs of DKA

Signs of DKA often reflect a sudden and significant decline and may worsen quickly without treatment. Signs may include:

- **Vomiting:** This is a hallmark sign of DKA and commonly associated with ketone buildup. Vomiting may be persistent.
- **Decreased appetite or refusal to eat:** Many cats stop eating entirely, due to nausea and discomfort.
- **Lethargy or weakness:** Cats may appear profoundly tired, weak, or unwilling to move.
- **Increased drinking and urination:** These are common early signs of diabetes and may still be present when DKA develops.
- **Dehydration:** Significant dehydration is common, despite increased drinking. See page 133 for Dehydration Assessment.
- **Weight loss:** Weight loss may occur rapidly.
- **Rapid or labored breathing:** Breathing may appear faster or deeper than normal.
- **Altered mental status or collapse:** Severe cases may cause disorientation, collapse, or minimal responsiveness.

What Can You Do?

Because the signs of diabetic ketoacidosis can overlap with many other serious conditions, prompt veterinary evaluation is important when changes in appetite, vomiting, drinking, urination, or behavior are noted.

- **Contact your veterinarian** promptly to discuss the signs and determine next steps.
  - If your veterinarian is unavailable, proceed to an **emergency veterinary facility.**
- **Minimize stress and handling.** Transport the cat in a secure carrier and keep them warm and calm during travel.
- **Know what is normal.** Being familiar with your cat's normal behaviors, drinking, urination, appetite, and energy levels can help identify concerning changes sooner.

Management of diabetic ketoacidosis is complex and intensive. Treatment typically requires hospitalization in a facility equipped for continuous monitoring and advanced supportive care.

At the veterinary clinic or hospital, you may expect the following:

- **Veterinary Examination**: A thorough physical exam will be performed, along with review of appetite changes, vomiting, drinking and urination patterns, insulin history if applicable, and any recent illness.
- **Blood Work and Urinalysis**: Blood tests and urinalysis are commonly performed to evaluate blood sugar levels, ketone presence, electrolyte status, and organ function.
- **IV Catheter Placement and Fluid Therapy:** An IV catheter will be placed early, and IV fluids will be started to address dehydration, support circulation, and help stabilize metabolic abnormalities.
- **Insulin Therapy:** Insulin is often administered as a continuous infusion with close monitoring. Blood sugar is checked frequently, and insulin dosing is adjusted carefully to allow safe stabilization.
- **Electrolyte Management:** Electrolyte imbalances are common in DKA and are monitored regularly and corrected as needed during treatment.
- **Evaluation for Concurrent Health Conditions:** Additional testing may be performed to identify infections or other diseases that may have contributed to the development of DKA.
- **Hospitalization:** Intensive monitoring, ongoing IV therapy, and repeated testing are typically required for several days.

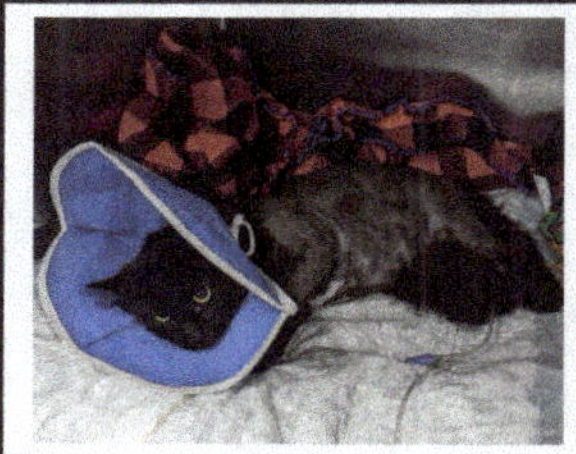

Figure 2.8. DKA is a true medical emergency requiring hospitalization and intensive veterinary care.

Photo credit: Dr. E Hampden-Smith

Prevention

Preventing diabetic ketoacidosis focuses on early recognition of diabetes, consistent management once diagnosed, and prompt response to illness.

- **Early recognition of diabetes**: Increased drinking and urination, weight loss, or appetite changes should prompt veterinary evaluation.
- **Consistent insulin use once diagnosed:** Missing insulin doses or changing dosing without guidance can increase the risk of DKA.
- **Consistent feeding schedule:** Diabetic cats are typically fed on a regular, often twice-daily, schedule alongside insulin. Changes in appetite or food intake should be addressed promptly.
- **Recognize warning signs of illness:** Vomiting, refusal to eat, lethargy, or sudden behavior changes warrant veterinary contact, especially in diabetic cats.
- **Routine veterinary care:** Regular rechecks help ensure insulin dosing is appropriate and complications are identified early.

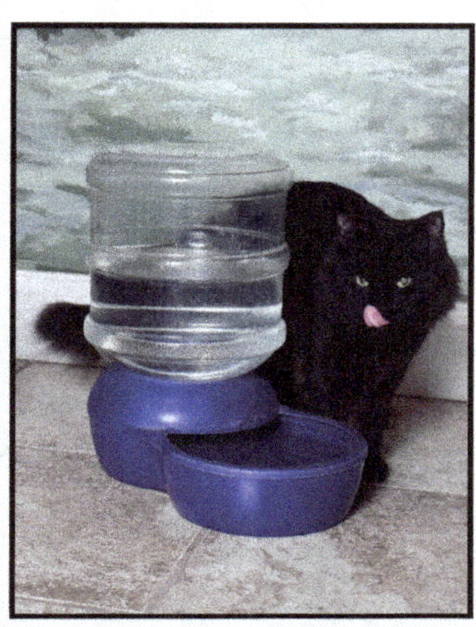

A Note About Diabetes

Diabetes mellitus is a condition in which the body cannot properly regulate blood sugar. The pancreas normally produces insulin, which allows sugar in the bloodstream to enter cells and be used for energy. When insulin is lacking or does not work effectively, blood sugar levels rise.

Most cats develop a form of diabetes similar to type 2 diabetes in people, involving insulin resistance and reduced insulin production. Some cats have more severe insulin deficiency, but most diabetic cats require insulin therapy to safely control blood sugar.

After Diagnosis:

- <u>Insulin is usually required.</u> Most cats need insulin at diagnosis to control blood sugar and prevent complications such as diabetic ketoacidosis.
- <u>Diet supports treatment but is not sufficient alone.</u> Nutrition and weight management are important, but diet alone is not a reliable or safe substitute for insulin.
- <u>Remission is possible for some cats.</u> With early diagnosis and appropriate treatment, some cats may enter diabetic remission.
  - Many cats remain insulin dependent long term. If remission does not occur, ongoing insulin therapy is often required.

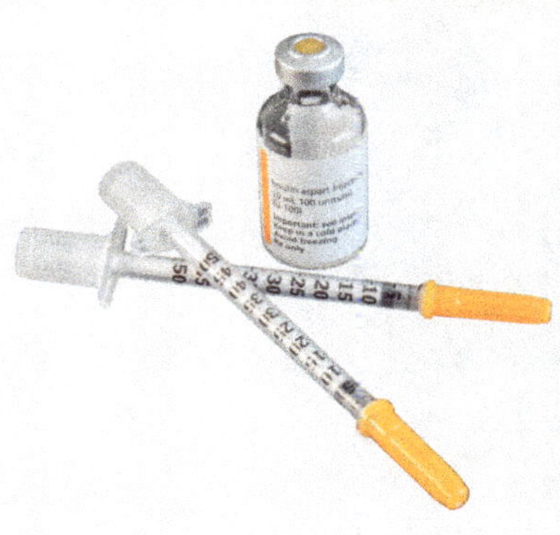

CONSTIPATION

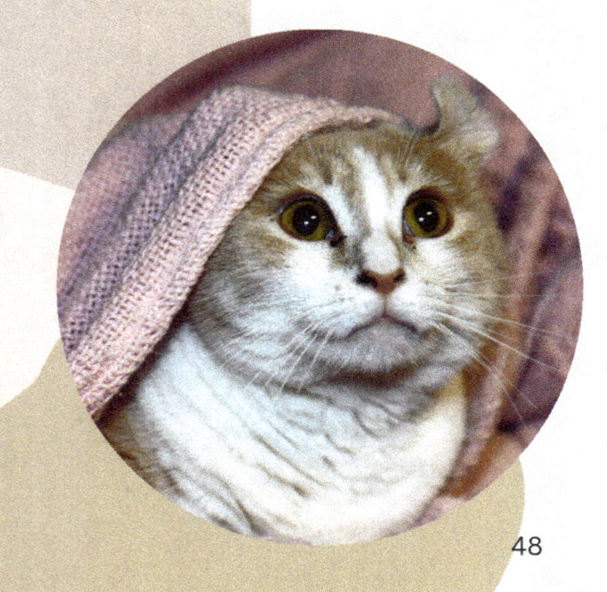

Possible Emergency

What is Constipation?

Constipation occurs when stool becomes difficult or painful to pass and accumulates in the colon. As stool sits in the colon, water continues to be absorbed, causing it to become dry, hard, and increasingly difficult to pass.

In more severe cases, constipation can progress to obstipation, where stool cannot be passed at all. Chronic or repeated constipation may eventually lead to megacolon, a condition in which the colon becomes abnormally enlarged and loses normal function.

Constipation can cause significant discomfort and, when severe or prolonged, may require medical intervention.

Cats Most Affected

Constipation can occur in cats of any age, but it is more commonly seen in:

- Middle-aged and senior cats
- Cats with chronic dehydration or kidney disease
- Overweight or obese cats
- Cats with arthritis, mobility limitations, or spinal disease
- Cats with a history of constipation or megacolon
- Manx cats and cats with congenital spinal abnormalities

Previous episodes of constipation increase the risk for future episodes.

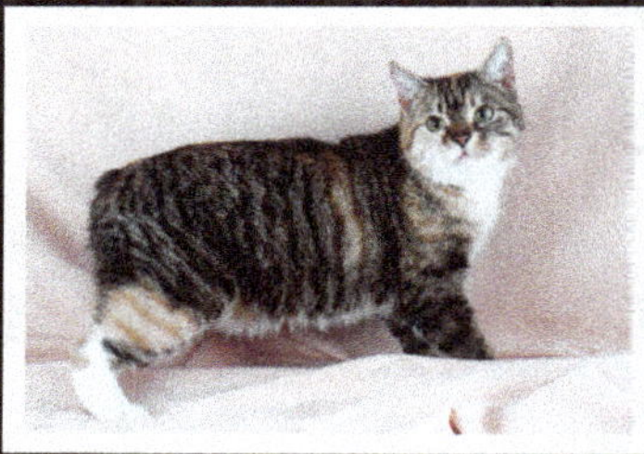

Manx cats have a naturally shortened or absent tail. Some have associated spinal abnormalities that can interfere with normal bowel function, increasing the risk of constipation.

Signs of Constipation

Signs of constipation may develop gradually or appear suddenly and can worsen if stool continues to accumulate. Signs may include:

- **Reduced or absent bowel movements:** Little to no stool passed for several days is common with constipation.
- **Straining to defecate:** Cats may make repeated, unproductive attempts to pass stool and may vocalize or appear uncomfortable.
- **Passing small, hard stools**: When stool is passed, it may be dry, firm, or pellet-like.
- **Vomiting:** Vomiting may occur, especially with more severe or prolonged constipation.
- **Decreased appetite**: Many cats eat less or stop eating altogether.
- **Lethargy:** Cats may appear tired, uncomfortable, or less interactive.
- **Abdominal discomfort**: Pain or sensitivity may be noted when the abdomen is touched.
- **Behavioral changes:** Hiding, irritability, or changes in litter box habits may occur.

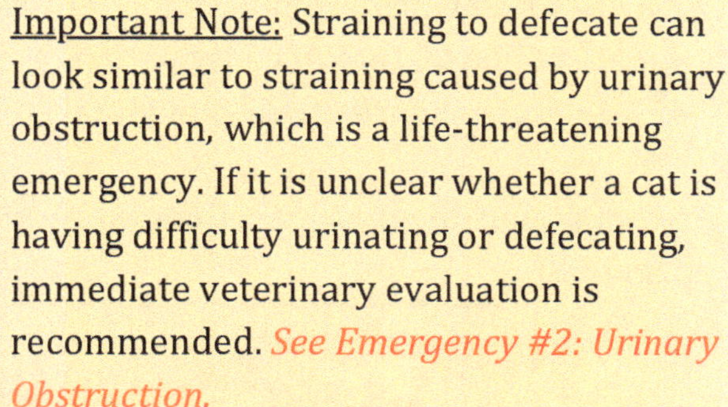

Important Note: Straining to defecate can look similar to straining caused by urinary obstruction, which is a life-threatening emergency. If it is unclear whether a cat is having difficulty urinating or defecating, immediate veterinary evaluation is recommended. *See Emergency #2: Urinary Obstruction.*

What Can You Do?

If you are concerned about your cat's defecation behavior and notice changes such as straining, reduced bowel movements, vomiting, or discomfort, veterinary evaluation is recommended.

- **Contact your veterinarian** promptly to discuss the signs and determine next steps.
  - If your veterinarian is unavailable, proceed to an urgent care or emergency veterinary facility.
  - **If you are unsure whether your cat has urinated,** seek emergency care immediately, as the signs of urinary obstruction and constipation can appear similar.
- **Minimize stress and handling:** Transport your cat in a secure carrier and keep them calm during travel.
- **Avoid home treatments** unless directed: Do not give over-the-counter laxatives, enemas, or human medications unless instructed by a veterinarian.

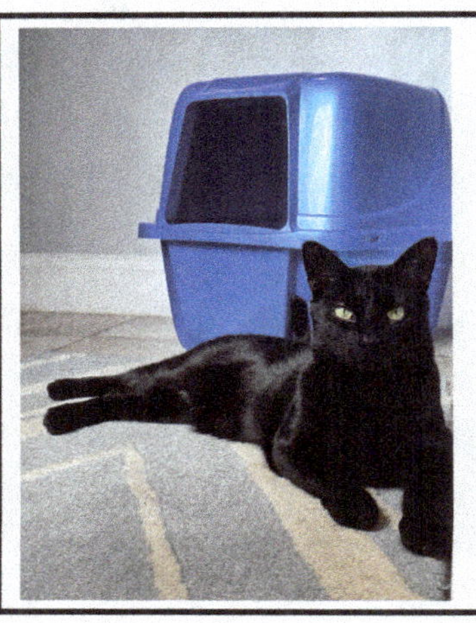

Monitoring litter box habits is important. Increased time in the box, discomfort, vocalization, or behavior changes may signal a medical concern.

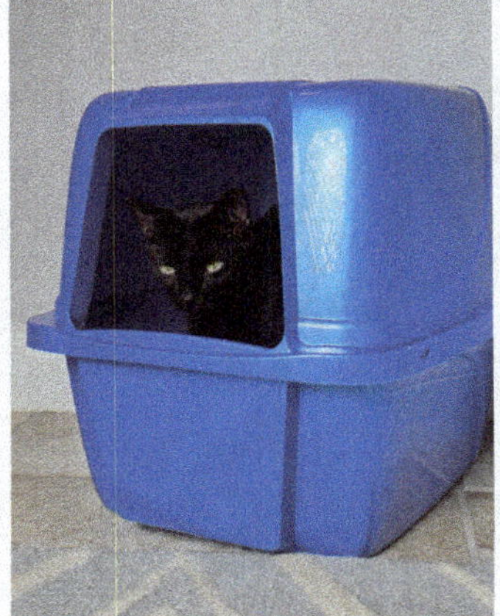

At the veterinary clinic or hospital, you may expect the following:

- **Veterinary Examination:** A physical exam will be performed, along with discussion of bowel movement history, diet, hydration, and recent behavior.

- **Diagnostic Testing:** Blood work may be used to assess hydration, kidney function, and electrolytes.
    - X-rays are commonly performed to evaluate stool burden, colon size, and contributing causes (see Fig. 2.9).

- **Fluid Therapy:** Dehydration is common and may be corrected with subcutaneous or intravenous fluids.

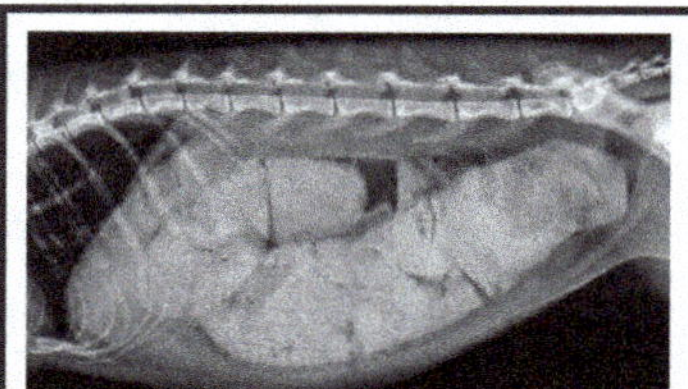

Figure 2.9. X-ray image showing a large amount of fecal material accumulated in the colon, consistent with constipation

Photo credit: Dr. M Meyer

- **Medications:** Stool softeners, laxatives, or medications to improve colonic movement may be prescribed once hydration is addressed.

- **Enemas:** Moderate to severe cases may require enemas using products that are safe for cats.

- **Manual Stool Removal:** Rarely, severe impaction may require removal under sedation or anesthesia if other treatments are unsuccessful.

- **Hospitalization:** Cats with significant impaction or dehydration may benefit from hospitalization for ongoing fluids and care, which may include repeated stool-softening treatments or delivery of solutions through a temporary feeding tube.

Constipation is not always preventable, but the following steps may help reduce risk:

- **Support hydration**: Encourage water intake by offering fresh water in multiple locations, using wide bowls or water fountains, and feeding canned food when appropriate.
- **Regular veterinary checkups**: Ongoing care helps identify medical conditions, such as kidney disease or electrolyte abnormalities, that may contribute to constipation.
  - As cats get older, more frequent visits are often recommended, sometimes twice yearly.
- **Promote healthy litter box access:** Ensure litter boxes are easy to enter, kept clean, and placed in quiet, low-stress locations, especially for older cats or those with mobility issues.
- **Address mobility and pain:** Cats with arthritis or chronic pain may avoid the litter box. Pain management and environmental adjustments can help maintain normal bowel habits.
- **Manage weight and activity:** Maintaining a healthy body condition and encouraging regular movement can support normal intestinal motility.
- **Monitor cats with prior constipation:** Cats with previous episodes are at higher risk for recurrence and may benefit from ongoing dietary or medical management as recommended by a veterinarian.

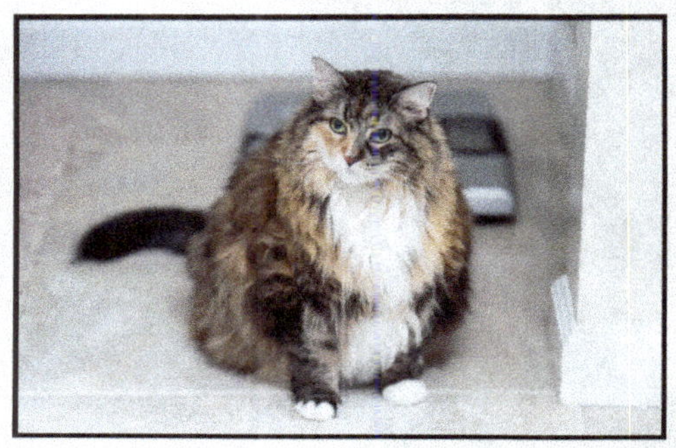

UPPER RESPIRATORY INFECTION

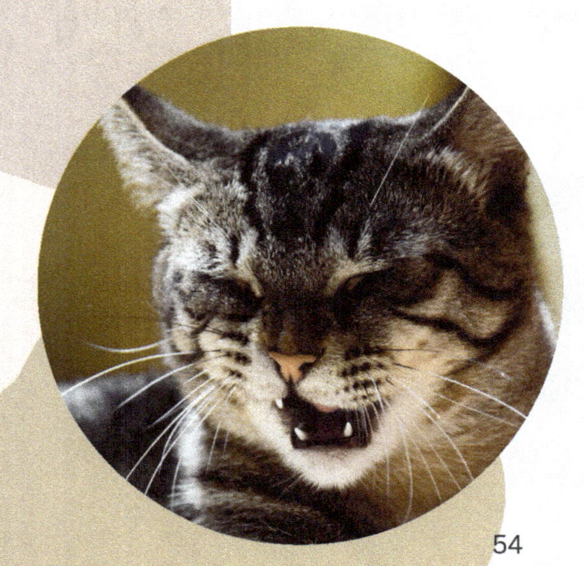

URI

Urgent

What is Upper Respiratory Infection (URI)?

Upper respiratory infections (URIs) are very common in cats, especially kittens. They affect the nose, eyes, mouth, and upper airways and are most often caused by viruses, particularly feline herpesvirus and feline calicivirus.

Stress can trigger illness or flare-ups, even in cats that previously appeared healthy. While many URIs are mild, some cases can become more serious, especially in young kittens, senior cats, or cats with underlying health conditions.

Cats Most Affected

Upper respiratory infections can occur in any cat, but some are at higher risk for developing illness or more severe signs:

- **Kittens:** Immature immune systems make kittens especially vulnerable and illness can progress quickly.
- **Senior cats:** Older cats may have reduced immune function or underlying disease that complicates recovery.
- **Cats from multi-cat environments:** Shelters, rescues, boarding facilities, and multi-cat households increase exposure risk.
- **Unvaccinated or under-vaccinated cats:** Vaccination does not prevent infection entirely but helps reduce severity.
- **Cats experiencing stress:** Recent moves, boarding, illness, surgery, or the introduction of a new pet can trigger illness or flare-ups.
- **Cats with underlying health conditions:** Immune compromise, chronic illness, or poor nutrition can worsen disease severity.

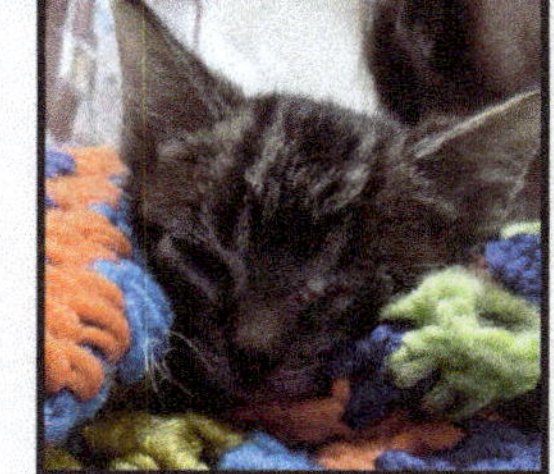

Photo credit: Dr. J. McCarthy

Signs of an upper respiratory infection may develop gradually or appear suddenly and often involve the eyes, nose, and mouth. Signs may include:

- **Sneezing:** Frequent or repetitive sneezing is common.
- **Nasal discharge:** Discharge may be clear, cloudy, yellow, or green.
  - **Congestion** or noisy breathing: Cats may sound "stuffy" or breathe noisily through the nose.
- **Eye discharge or redness:** Watery or thick discharge, squinting, or swollen eyelids may be seen.

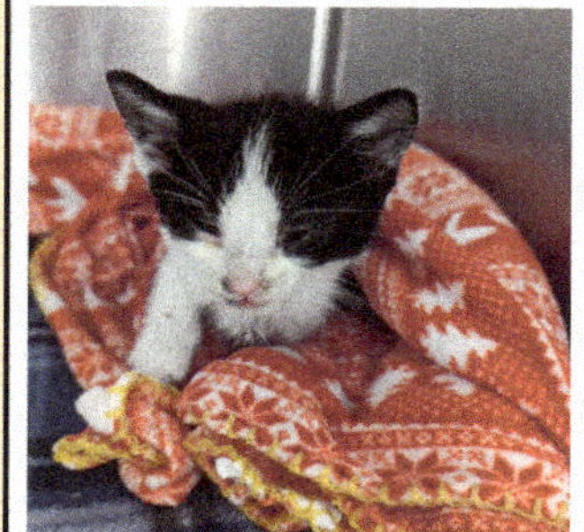

Figure 2.10. Nasal congestion and discharge, along with eye discharge, are very common signs of URIs.

Photo credit: Dr. E. Hampden-Smith

- **Decreased appetite**: Loss of smell from nasal congestion often leads to reduced interest in food.
- **Lethargy:** Cats may appear tired, less interactive, or withdrawn.
- **Mouth or tongue ulcers:** These are more commonly seen with calicivirus and may cause drooling or pain when eating.

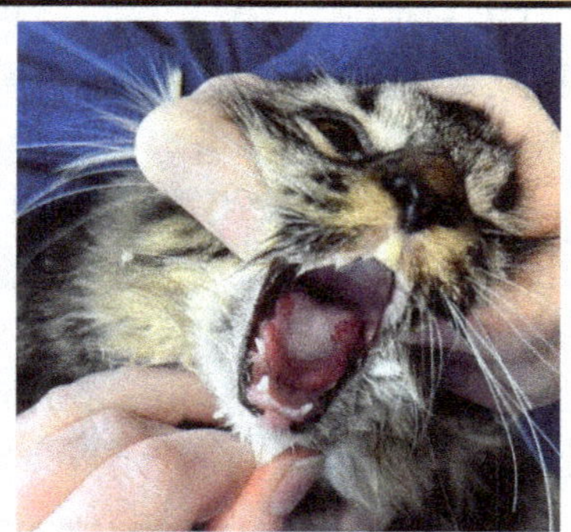

Figure 2.11. Ulcerations of the tongue and mouth are possible with URIs. They can be quite painful and require veterinary care.

Photo credit: Dr. K. Neff

If you notice signs of an upper respiratory infection, veterinary evaluation is recommended to assess severity and determine next steps.

Contact your veterinarian to discuss the signs and schedule an appointment. Many cats with mild symptoms can be managed on an outpatient basis.

- **Seek urgent or emergency care** if your cat stops eating or drinking, appears dehydrated, has difficulty breathing, or becomes markedly lethargic.
- **Minimize stress:** Keep your cat in a quiet, warm environment and avoid unnecessary handling as stress can worsen symptoms.
- **Encourage food and water intake:** Strong-smelling foods and warmed meals may help stimulate appetite.
- **Humidified air:** Brief exposure to humid air (such as sitting in a steamy bathroom) can help loosen nasal secretions and improve comfort in congested cats.

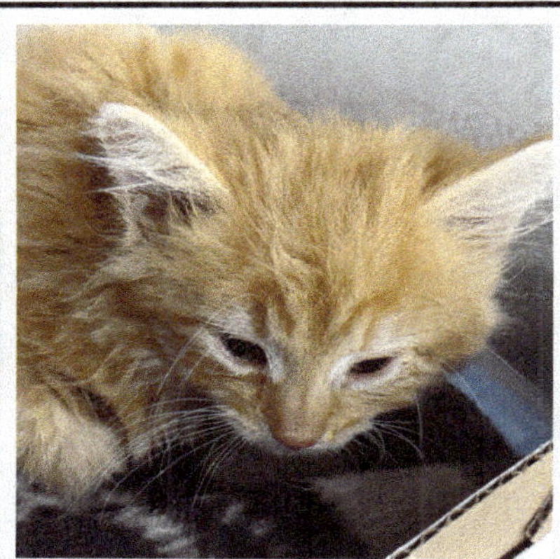

Figure 2.12. URIs can be seen in any cat. However, kittens are especially predisposed due to their immature immune systems.

Photo credit: Dr. E. Hampden-Smith

A Note About Nasal Congestion and Respiratory Distress

Nasal congestion can make cats sound uncomfortable and may occasionally cause brief open-mouth breathing. This does not always mean your cat is in respiratory distress. However, it can be difficult to tell the difference and careful observation is important.

If you are unsure whether congestion is affecting breathing, you can try the following:

- **Gently clear the nostrils:**
  - If nasal discharge is crusted or blocking the nostrils, use a warm, damp washcloth to gently wipe the area and improve airflow.
- **Check resting respiratory rate:**
  - Count breaths while your cat is resting or sleeping. A normal resting respiratory rate is typically under 40 breaths per minute. More details on how to check this are covered in your Emergency Toolkit (Chapter 4, page 110).
- **Watch for breathing effort:**
  - Breathing should appear smooth and quiet. Increased abdominal movement, exaggerated chest motion, or visible effort are more concerning signs.
- **Try humidified air:**
  - If your cat seems otherwise comfortable, sitting with them in a steamy bathroom for several minutes may help loosen nasal congestion and improve comfort.

If your cat appears distressed, is breathing with effort, or you are unsure whether breathing is normal, the safest choice is to trust your instincts and seek veterinary care promptly.

At a veterinary facility, common interventions for URIs may include:

- **Veterinary examination:** A thorough physical exam will be performed. Because upper respiratory infections are often contagious between cats, your cat may be examined or housed in an isolation area to protect other patients.
- **Medications** (when indicated):
  - Antibiotics may be prescribed if there is concern for secondary bacterial infection. Antiviral medications may be recommended in more severe or prolonged cases. Eye medications may be prescribed when secondary conjunctivitis is present.
- **Supportive care:** Many cats are managed at home with supportive care focused on comfort, hydration, and maintaining appetite while the immune system clears the infection.
- **Hospitalization:** Hospitalization is rarely needed but may be recommended for cats that are not eating or drinking, are significantly dehydrated, or have breathing concerns.

Most uncomplicated upper respiratory infections improve with time and supportive care, but veterinary guidance helps ensure complications are identified early.

Prevention

Upper respiratory infections are not always preventable. The following steps may help reduce risk and severity:
- **Vaccination:** This helps reduce severity and duration of illness.
- **Stress reduction:** Stress can trigger illness, especially in herpesvirus carriers.
- **Limit exposure:** Avoid contact with sick cats.
- **Overall health support:** Good nutrition, hydration, and regular veterinary checkups support immune function.

SEVERE ANEMIA

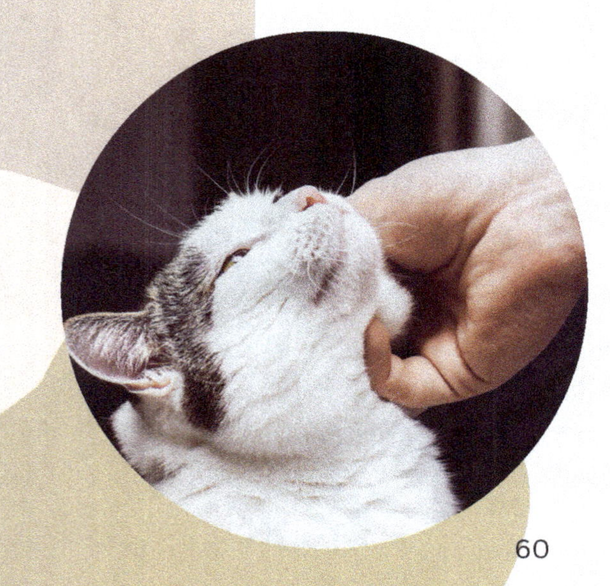

What is Significant Anemia?

Significant anemia occurs when a cat has a critically low number of red blood cells, reducing the body's ability to deliver oxygen to tissues. When severe, anemia can quickly lead to weakness, collapse, and organ dysfunction.

Anemia is described as a dangerous reduction in red blood cells rather than a specific diagnosis. It develops as a result of an underlying problem, such as blood loss, red blood cell destruction, or decreased red blood cell production.

Cats often hide illness well, so signs may be subtle until anemia becomes advanced. Prompt veterinary evaluation is essential once anemia is suspected.

Common Causes of Significant Anemia

Severe anemia can develop for a variety of reasons. Common causes in cats include:

- **Parasites:**
  - External parasites (especially fleas) and internal parasites can cause blood loss, especially in young kittens or small cats.
- **Chronic kidney disease:**
  - The kidneys produce erythropoietin (EPO), a hormone that signals the body to make red blood cells. With kidney disease, reduced EPO production leads to anemia over time.
- **Immune-mediated hemolytic anemia (IMHA):**
  - In IMHA, the immune system destroys red blood cells. This may occur without an identifiable trigger (idiopathic) or be associated with underlying conditions such as cancer, infections, inflammation, or medications.
- **Blood loss:**
  - Trauma, internal bleeding, clotting disorders, or gastrointestinal bleeding can lead to acute or progressive anemia.

Severe anemia can occur in cats of any age, but certain cats are at higher risk:

- **Cats with immune-mediated disease,** including immune-mediated destruction of red blood cells
- **Cats with chronic illness,** such as kidney disease, cancer, or inflammatory conditions
- **Cats exposed to toxins or medications** that damage red blood cells or interfere with production
- **Cats with parasitic disease,** including severe flea infestations (more common in kittens or unprotected cats)

Anemia may develop suddenly or worsen quietly over time, making early recognition challenging.

Signs of Severe Anemia

Signs of severe anemia often reflect decreased oxygen delivery to the body and may worsen rapidly. Signs may include:

- **Lethargy or weakness:** Cats may appear unusually tired, reluctant to move, or unable to jump or walk normally.
- **Decreased appetite**: Reduced interest in food is common.
- **Pale or white gums**: When the lip is gently lifted, gum color may appear lighter than normal (See Figure 2.14).
- **Rapid breathing or breathing with exertion**: Breathing may become rapid, even when the cat is at rest.
- **Collapse or extreme weakness:** In severe cases, cats may collapse or be unable to stand.
- **Hiding or decreased interaction:** Many cats withdraw or isolate themselves when unwell.
- **Yellow discoloration of the gums, eyes, or ears:** This may be seen in cases involving red blood cell destruction (See Figure 2.13).

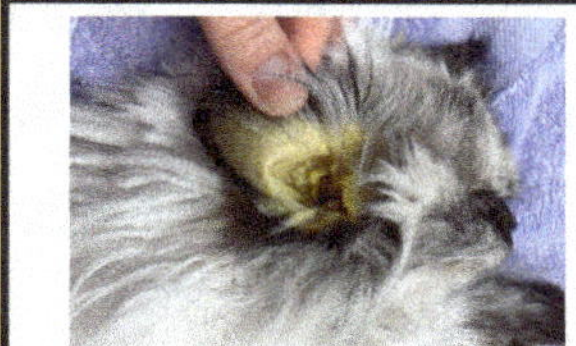

Figure 2.13. Yellow discoloration of the skin is a concerning sign that requires veterinary assessment.
Photo credit Dr. Jones Cross

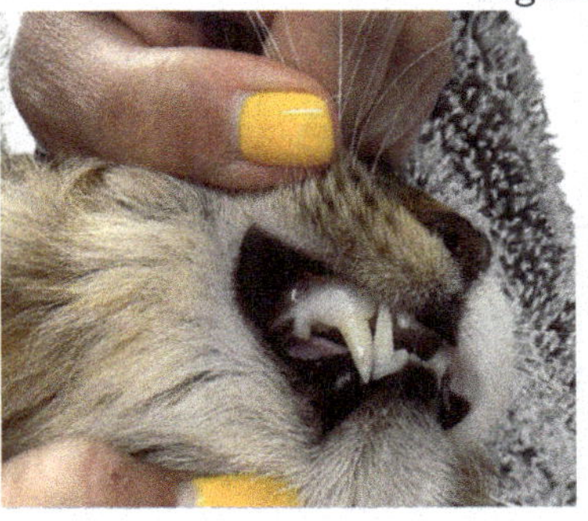

A photograph demonstrating
pale gums

Photo credit: Dr. E. Leaf Jennings

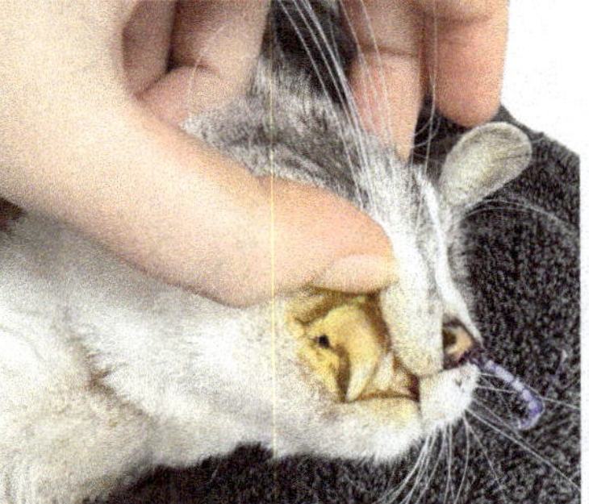

A photograph demonstrating
yellow (jaundiced) gums

Photo credit: Dr K. Hutton

What Can You Do?

Changes in energy, appetite, or behavior should prompt veterinary evaluation, as these may be early signs of illness, including anemia. Cats often compensate well until disease becomes advanced, so subtle changes should not be ignored.

Certain findings are more emergent. Pale or white gums, rapid breathing while at rest, marked weakness, or collapse indicate reduced oxygen delivery and warrant immediate veterinary or emergency care.

- **Contact your veterinarian promptly** to discuss concerning changes and determine next steps.
- **Seek emergency care immediately** if pale gums, rapid breathing at rest, weakness, or collapse are noted.
- **Minimize stress and handling:** Keep the cat calm, warm, and in a secure carrier during transport, and avoid unnecessary exertion.

Early evaluation can be lifesaving when anemia is severe.

At a veterinary facility, common interventions for severe anemia may include:

- **Veterinary examination:** A focused physical exam will assess gum color, heart rate, breathing pattern, and overall stability.
- **Bloodwork:** Blood tests are used to confirm anemia, assess severity, and provide clues about possible causes (such as blood loss, red blood cell destruction, or decreased production).
- **Additional diagnostics:** Depending on initial findings, testing may include blood smear evaluation, imaging (X-rays and/or abdominal ultrasound), infectious disease testing, clotting tests, or other specialized diagnostics as needed.
- **Oxygen support:** Supplemental oxygen may be provided if anemia is causing breathing difficulty or weakness.
- **Blood transfusion:** In cases of severe or rapidly worsening anemia, a blood transfusion may be necessary to stabilize the cat.
- **Treatment of the underlying cause:** This may include medications, parasite treatment, management of bleeding, or therapy directed at immune-mediated disease or toxins.
- **Hospitalization:** Cats with significant anemia are often hospitalized for close monitoring and supportive care while treatment is initiated. Hospitalization may be prolonged.

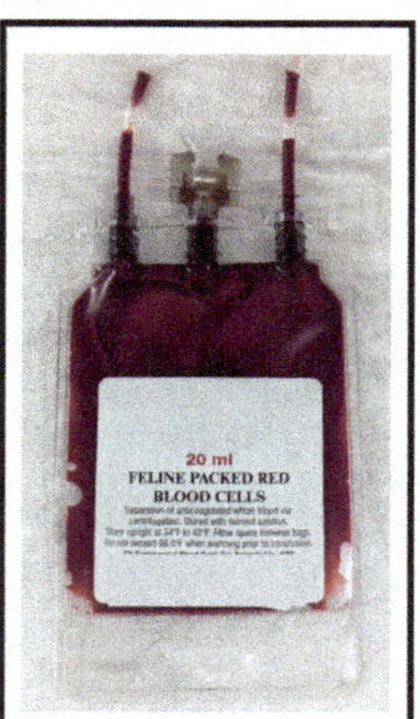

Blood transfusions are often needed if anemia is severe.

Severe anemia requires prompt veterinary care. Early stabilization and identification of the cause are critical for recovery.

Prevention

Severe anemia is not always preventable, but the following steps may help reduce risk and support early identification:

- **Routine veterinary care:** Regular wellness visits help detect anemia early, especially in senior cats or those with chronic conditions. As cats age, visits are often recommended twice yearly.
- **Parasite prevention:** Consistent flea prevention is important, particularly for kittens or cats in flea-endemic areas, as heavy infestations can lead to significant blood loss.
- **Toxin awareness:** Familiarity with common household and environmental toxins, including rodenticides and certain medications, helps reduce accidental exposure. See Chapter 3 for a listing of the ten most common toxicities.
  - Keep the pet poison control phone number readily available.
  - **ASPCA Poison Control: (888) 426-4435** (USA and Canada)
- **Medication caution**: Medications should only be given under veterinary guidance, as some drugs can contribute to anemia or bleeding.

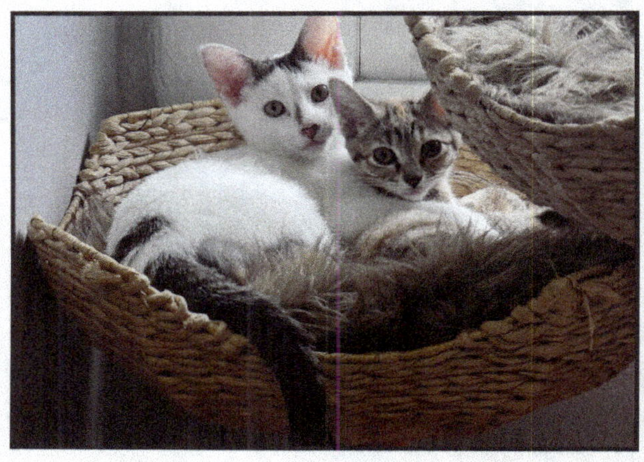

TRAUMA

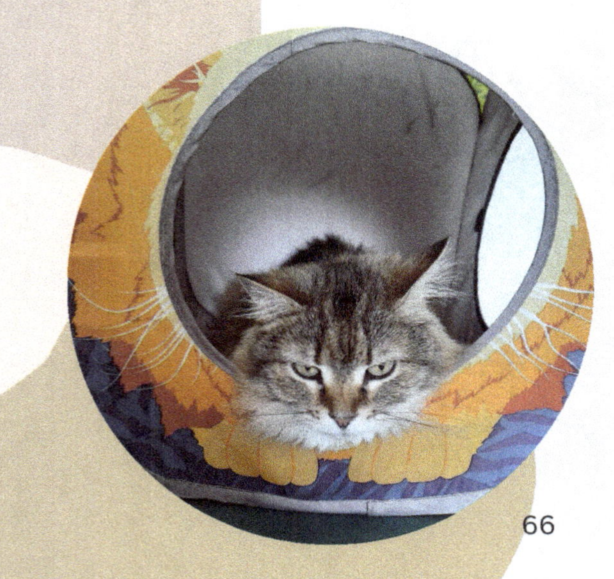

Possible Emergency

What is Trauma?

Trauma in cats refers to physical injury caused by accidents, falls, animal attacks, or vehicle collisions. Injuries can range from superficial wounds to serious internal damage requiring immediate veterinary care.

Because cats often hide pain and injury, trauma may be more severe than it initially appears. Signs of serious injury are not always obvious, and even seemingly minor incidents can result in life-threatening complications.

Additional guidance on recognizing emergency warning signs is covered in Chapter Four.

Cats Most Affected

Trauma can affect any cat, but increased risk is seen in:
- Cats with outdoor access or that escape outdoors
- Cats living in multi-story homes or apartments (because of falls from height)
- Young, curious cats and kittens

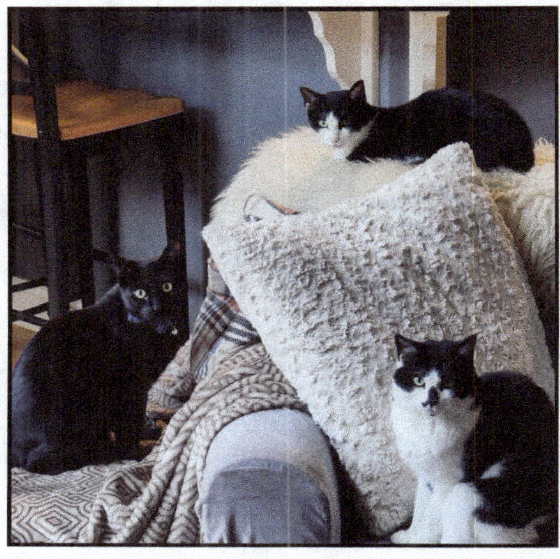

Signs of Trauma

Signs of trauma in cats may be obvious or subtle. Any of the following should be taken seriously:

- **Limping or reluctance to move**: Difficulty walking, stiffness, hiding, or refusing to move can indicate pain, fractures, or internal injury.
- **Visible wounds, swelling, or bruising:** Bite wounds, punctures, scrapes, swelling, or blood noted on the fur or skin are concerning, even if injuries appear minor.
- **Altered mentation:** Disorientation, unresponsiveness, collapse, or unusual behavior can suggest head injury or shock.
- **Pain-related behaviors:** Hiding, growling, hissing, vocalizing, or sudden aggression may be signs of significant pain.
- **Breathing changes:** Rapid breathing, open-mouth breathing, or increased effort at rest are urgent warning signs.

Because cats often mask pain and injury, trauma may be more severe than it appears. When in doubt, veterinary evaluation is recommended.

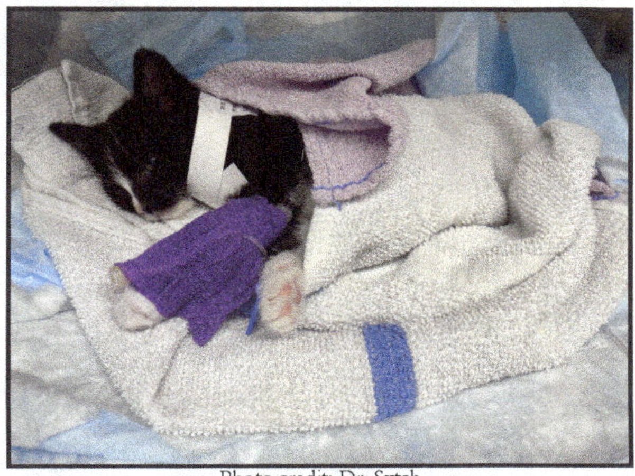

Photo credit: Dr. Sytch

If a cat experiences trauma, the safest approach is to assume injuries may be more serious than they appear.

- **Minimize movement:** Keep the cat confined to a small, quiet space or carrier. Avoid jumping, running, or stairs.
- **Handle with care:** Cats may react unpredictably when injured. Use a towel or blanket if needed and avoid excessive handling.

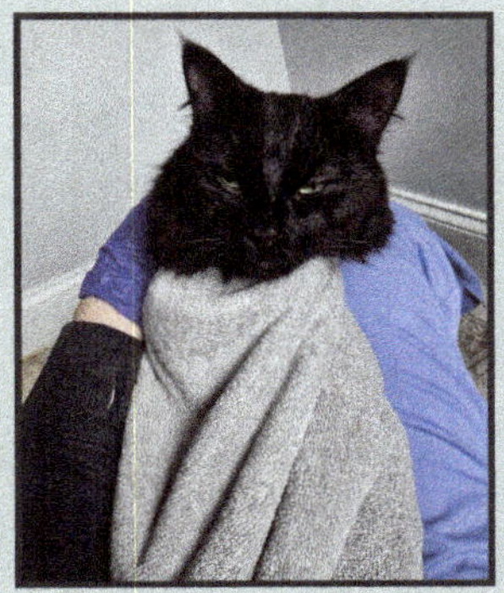

- **<u>Do not attempt home treatment:</u>** Do not give medications or attempt to clean deep wounds at home, as either may worsen injuries or delay care.
- **Contact a veterinarian promptly:** Even if injuries seem minor, veterinary guidance is important after trauma.

Seek *immediate* emergency care if any of the following are noted:

- Difficulty breathing or rapid breathing at rest
- Collapse, weakness, or inability to stand
- Pale gums or altered responsiveness
- Suspected high-impact injury (a fall from height, vehicle strike, or animal attack)

During transport, keep the cat calm, warm, and secure in a carrier, and limit movement as much as possible.

Note: Some trauma-related complications, including breathing difficulties, may develop hours to days after the injury. Close monitoring is needed!

While each case is different, here are some common interventions relative to trauma that are to be expected at the veterinary hospital, depending on each cat's needs:

- **Veterinary examination:** A thorough physical examination is performed to assess pain, visible injuries, breathing, circulation, and overall stability.
- **Stabilization:** Supportive care such as IV fluids, oxygen therapy, and temperature support may be provided if shock or respiratory compromise is present.
- **Diagnostic testing:** Blood work and diagnostic imaging (such as X-rays or ultrasound) may be performed to evaluate for internal injuries, fractures, or bleeding.
- **Pain management:** Pain medications are administered to improve comfort and reduce stress.
- **Wound care:** Wounds may be cleaned, flushed, sutured, or otherwise managed to reduce the risk of infection.
- **Surgery:** Surgical intervention may be required for internal injuries, fractures, or significant wounds.

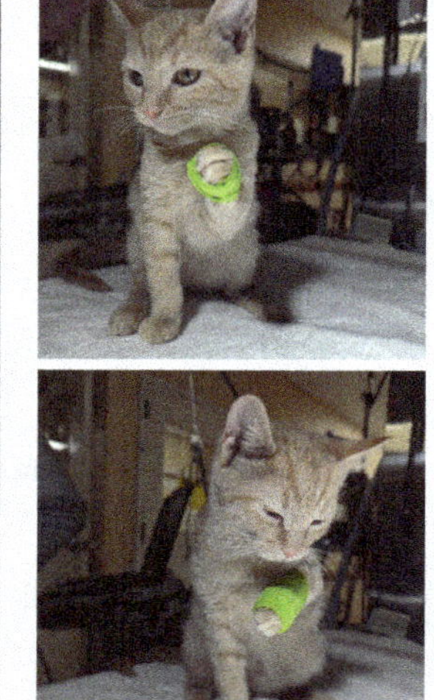

Figure 2.15. Bandaging may be performed to cover a wound or control bleeding.

- **Neurologic assessment:** A neurologic examination may be performed if head trauma or spinal injury is suspected.
- **Hospitalization and monitoring:** Ongoing hospitalization may be recommended to monitor breathing and control pain and response to treatment, as some complications can develop over time.

Not all trauma can be prevented, but the following steps may help reduce risk:

- **Window and balcony safety:** Secure windows, screens, and balconies to reduce the risk of falls, especially in multi-story homes.
- **Safe transport**: Transport cats in a secure carrier to reduce the risk of injury or escape during travel.
- **Outdoor safety considerations:** Outdoor access increases the risk of vehicle injury, animal encounters, and falls. Keeping cats indoors is the safest option; however, if outdoor access is chosen, extra awareness of these risks is important. 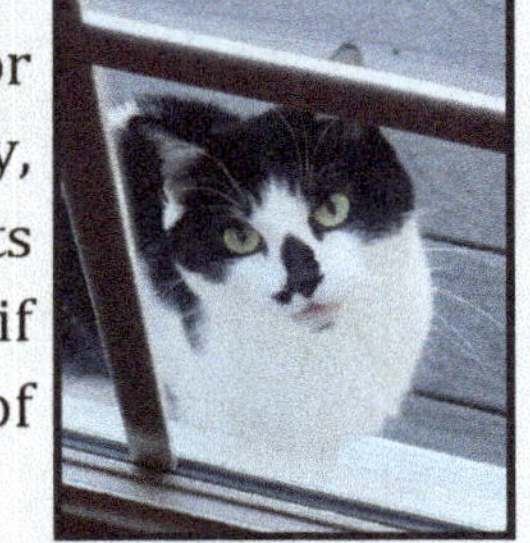
- **Environmental awareness:** Be mindful of household hazards such as recliners, garage doors, washing machines, and dryers, which can cause accidental injury.
- **Conflict reduction:** In multi-pet households, thoughtful introductions and management of known aggression can help reduce fight-related injuries.
- **Prompt evaluation after injury:** Early veterinary assessment after trauma may help identify internal injuries before complications develop.

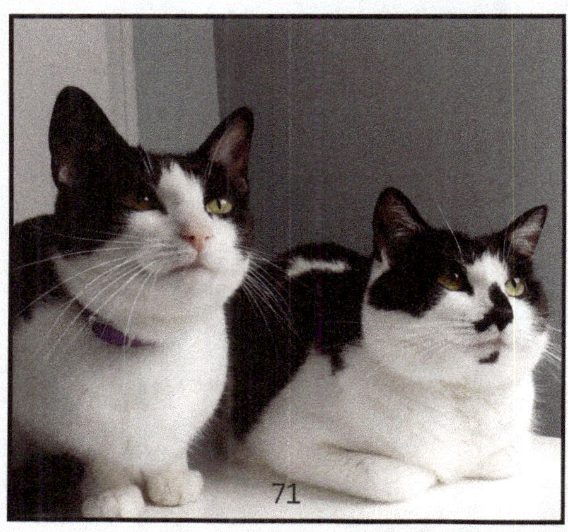

TEN MOST COMMON TOXICITIES

Because of cats' curious nature, exposure to toxic or potentially toxic substances is a common concern in veterinary medicine. Although many toxins exist, knowing the most common ones is important since faster response times can significantly affect outcomes.

Upon evaluating 12 months of data collected by ASPCA Poison Control in 2025, the top ten toxins will be discussed in this chapter.

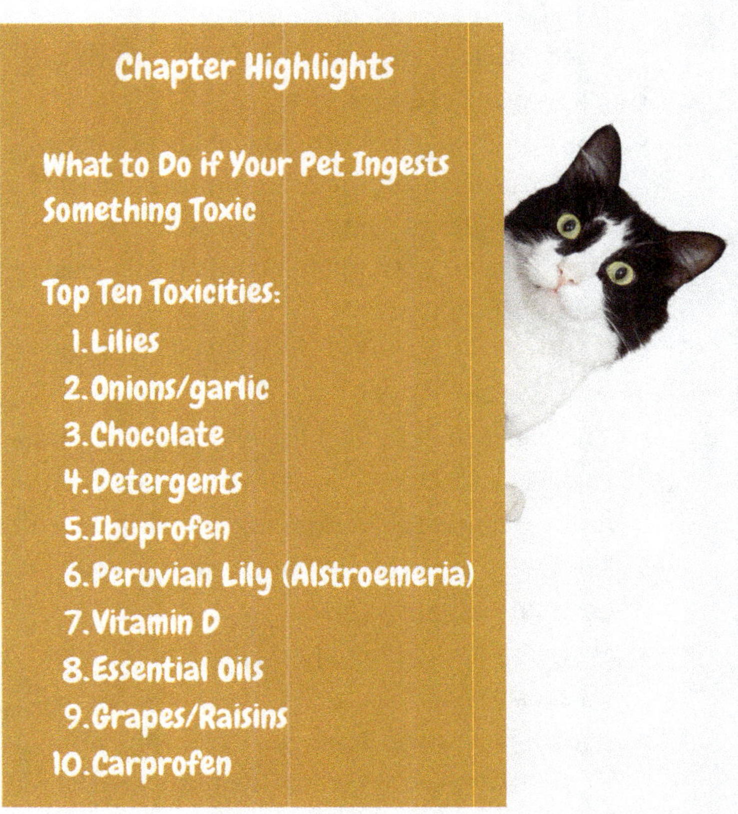

Note: Doses are generally calculated in mg/kg. That is the concentration of a medication/toxin in milligrams (mg) divided by the cat's weight in kilograms (kg).

To calculate your cat's weight in kg, simply divide their weight in pounds (lbs) by 2.2.
For example: a 10 pound cat / 2.2 = 4.5 kg

ASPCA Poison Control: (888) 426-4435

1. **Assess the situation and gather information.**
   - Identify **what** your cat ingested/ was exposed to.
     - If you have the packaging available, have it handy.
   - Identify **how much** was ingested.
   - Identify **when** the exposure occurred.
   - Have a rough idea of your cat's **weight.**
   - Keep track of any **clinical signs** you may be seeing.
2. **Contact your veterinarian.**
   - For mild toxicities with known products, your vet may be able to provide sufficient guidance for the best way to ensure your cat's safety. However, be aware that a consultation with poison control may still be needed.
3. **Contact Poison Control.**
   - **ASPCA Poison Control: (888) 426-4435**
     - Available 24/7
   - This service provides expert advice on what to do in any toxicity situation. They will discuss anything you can do at home or make recommendations for veterinary care.
   - They also provide guidance to any veterinarian who may be treating your cat.
   - You may opt to skip step 2 and call Poison Control directly!
4. **Follow instructions** from your veterinarian/Poison Control.
   - Do not attempt to intervene at home without guidance.
   - Do not attempt to induce vomiting at home! There is no safe way to do this with a cat.
5. **DO NOT wait for symptoms to be seen**.
   - It is important to act immediately.
   - The earlier you begin interventions, the better the outcome.

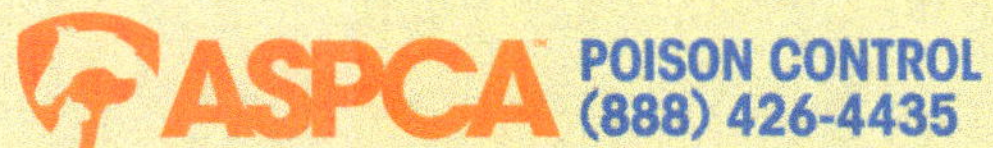

Some pet families are unclear about why we, as vets, recommend calling Poison Control for toxicities, as there is a fee associated with consultation. Here are some of the reasons why we do this:

- **Specialized Expertise**
  - Poison Control Centers are staffed by experts who specialize in toxicology and have access to extensive databases. They can provide the most accurate and up-to-date information regarding specific toxins and treatments.
- **24/7 Availability**
  - They operate around the clock, ensuring that pet owners can get immediate assistance any time of day.
- **Follow-Up Care**
  - They are available for follow-up if any questions should arise about the situation in the near future.
- **Comprehensive Resources**
  - They have access to a wide range of resources and protocols that may not be available to individual veterinarians, allowing them to provide tailored advice based on the specific situation your pet is handling.
- **Guidance with Next Steps**
  - They help pet owners determine whether a situation is an emergency and what immediate action to take, including any home remedies or the need for vet care.
  - Guidance regarding care is also provided to any veterinarian who is caring for your cat.
- **Cost Effectiveness**
  - While there is a fee, the expertise and immediate guidance offered can save pet owners from costly treatments or missteps.

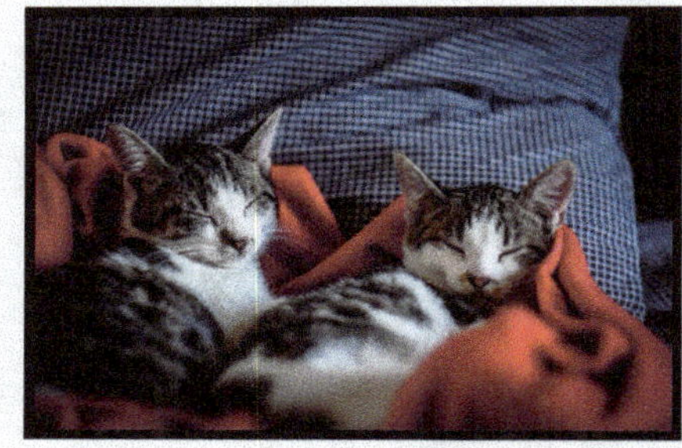

LILIES

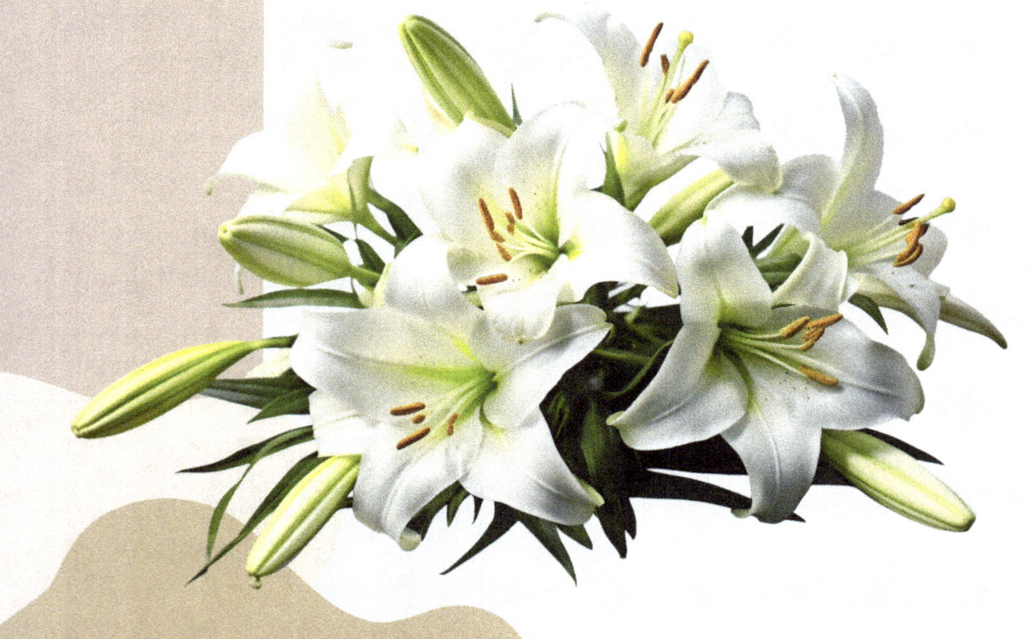

Lilies represent one of the most dangerous toxic exposures to cats and are a leading cause of emergency poison control calls. Exposure often occurs in subtle ways, such as contact with pollen, grooming contaminated fur, chewing plant material, or drinking vase water. Even minimal exposure can result in severe and rapidly progressive kidney failure.

The exact toxic compound in true lilies has not been definitively identified. What is known is that the toxin causes direct damage to kidney cells, leading to acute kidney failure.

Not all lilies affect the kidneys.

True lilies (*Lilium spp.*) and daylilies (*Hemerocallis spp.*) are uniquely toxic to cats, leading to kidney injury.

Other plants, such as Peruvian lilies (see toxicity #6), peace lilies, and calla lilies, do not cause kidney failure, though some may cause oral irritation or gastrointestinal upset.

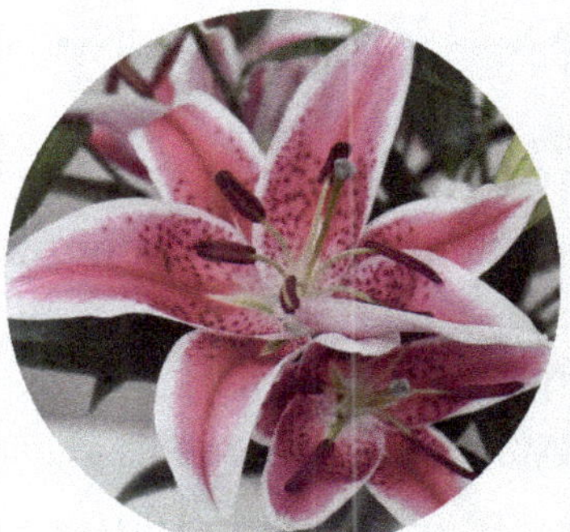

True Lily

Stargazer Lily, (*Lilium orientalis*)

Other Lilies- NOT Kidney Toxic

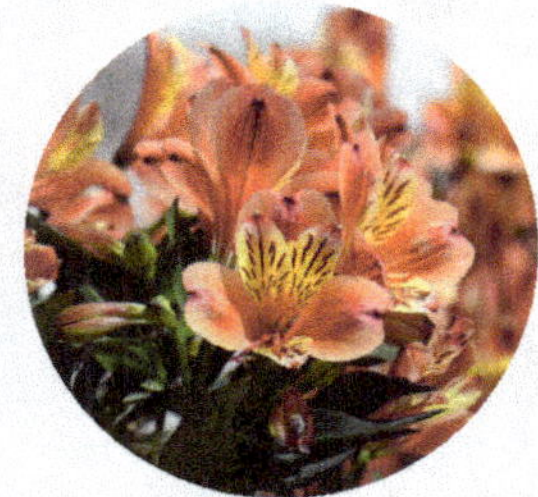

Peruvian Lily

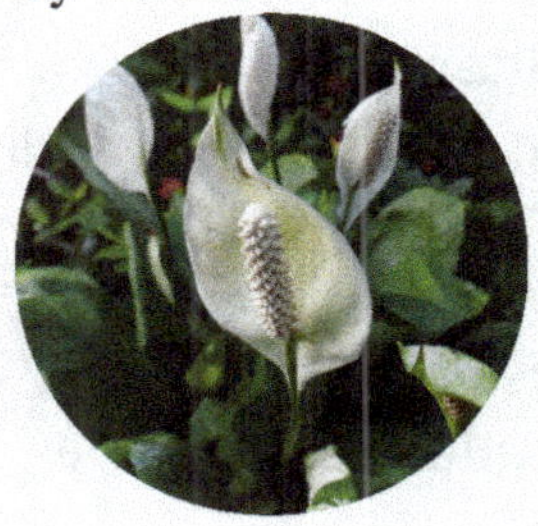

Peace Lily

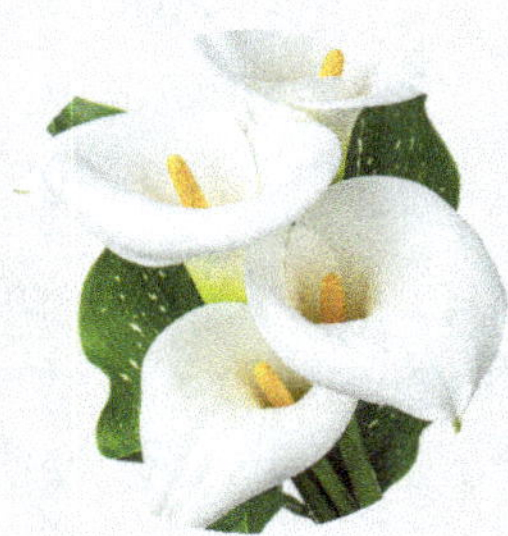

Calla Lily

<h1 style="text-align:center">Toxicity Level:</h1>

There is no known safe dose. Any exposure, including contact with pollen, rubbing against the plant, drinking from vase water, or ingestion of a small portion of the plant, should be considered an emergency.

Signs of Toxicity

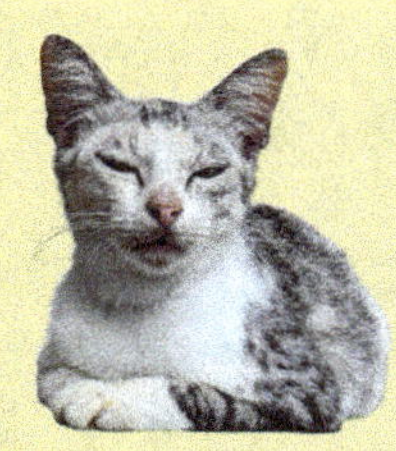

- **Initial Signs (sometimed delayed)**
  - Vomiting
  - Diarrhea
  - Lethargy
  - Loss of appetite

  Note: Delayed signs may be seen in the absence of early signs.
- **Delayed Signs (within 24 to 72 hours)**
  - Increased thirst and urination
  - Abdominal pain
  - Dehydration
  - Kidney failure
    - May be accompanied by decreased urination

Common Interventions

- Contact Poison Control to determine if veterinary care is needed.
- If a vet visit is recommended, common interventions may include the following:
  - Inducing Vomiting - depending on the timeline
  - Baseline Blood Work - especially to assess kidney values
  - Providing IV Fluids and Symptomatic Care - with medications to protect the gastrointestinal tract
  - Hospitalization - often for at least 48 hours
  - Ongoing Monitoring and Repeated Blood Work

Prognosis: With rapid intervention and absence of signs of kidney failure within 72 hours, the prognosis is very good. Prognosis becomes less favorable if kidney failure does occur.

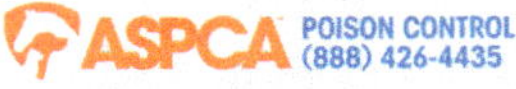

GARLIC/ ONION

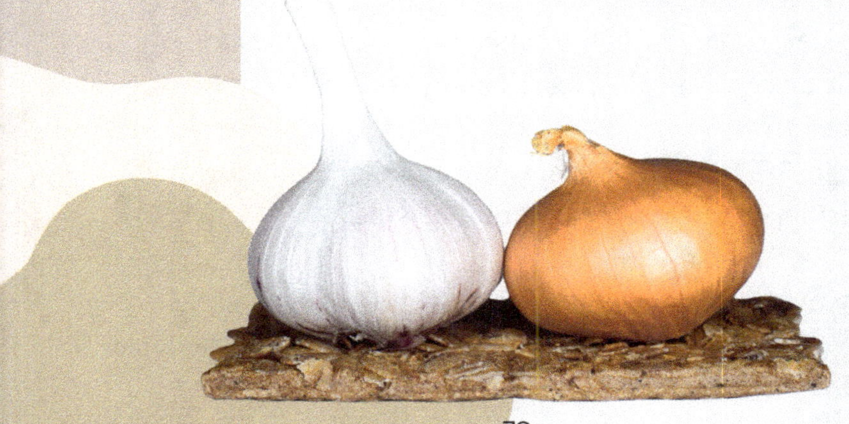

Common kitchen staples and garden vegetables like garlic and onions belong to the *Allium* family and contain toxins called disulfides, which can be harmful to cats, leading to gastrointestinal signs and anemia (see page 126). Cats appear more sensitive to the toxic effects than dogs.

Toxin: Disulfides

Disulfides can damage red blood cells, which may result in hemolytic anemia, where red blood cells are destroyed faster than they can be produced. Cats lack certain enzymes that help protect their red blood cells from the effects of disulfides, making them particularly vulnerable to its toxic effects.

Toxicity Level

Small exposures over a prolonged time can cause chronic anemia and signs. Caution should be exercised with feeding people-food (even baby food), which may contain onions or garlic.

- <u>Raw /Cooked Onion:</u> Clinical toxicity can occur from relatively small amounts. Cooking does not destroy the toxic compounds. Risk is highest with repeated exposure.
  - Concentration may increase or decrease depending on preparation method
- <u>Powdered Onion</u>: Highly concentrated and therefore more toxic per volume. Even small amounts used in seasoning can pose a risk.
- <u>Garlic:</u> 3-5 times more concentrated than onions. Not considered safe at any amount ingested!

MOST to LEAST

Toxicity may occur at 5g/kg of onions and 1g/kg of garlic. Repeated exposure to smaller doses can lead to clinical toxicity.

Signs of Toxicity

Signs of poisoning from onions, garlic, or chives may <u>not</u> appear immediately. In cats, signs may be seen in as few as 12 hours or may be delayed for multiple days.

- Vomiting: Cats may vomit shortly after ingestion, although signs are often delayed from time of ingestion.
- Diarrhea: This may accompany vomiting and can lead to dehydration.
- Lethargy: Affected cats may show signs of weakness and a general lack of energy.
- **Decrease in Red Blood Cells (Anemia).** Signs may include:
  - Pale gums
  - Increased heart rate
  - Weakness
  - Collapse
  - Rapid breathing
  - Discoloration of urine
  - Jaundice

Common Interventions

- Contact Animal Poison Control for guidance.
  - At-home monitoring is often recommended.
- If a veterinary visit is recommended, common interventions may include:
  - Monitoring Blood Work: This is typical at presentation and may then be repeated for approximately one week.
  - IV fluids may be administered as needed for dehydration.
  - Supportive Care: Oxygen therapy and blood transfusions may be administered as needed until the body can produce its own red cells.

Prognosis: With early identification and supportive care, the prognosis is generally good. Prognosis becomes more guarded in cases of significant anemia or delayed treatment.

ASPCA POISON CONTROL (888) 426-4435

CHOCOLATE

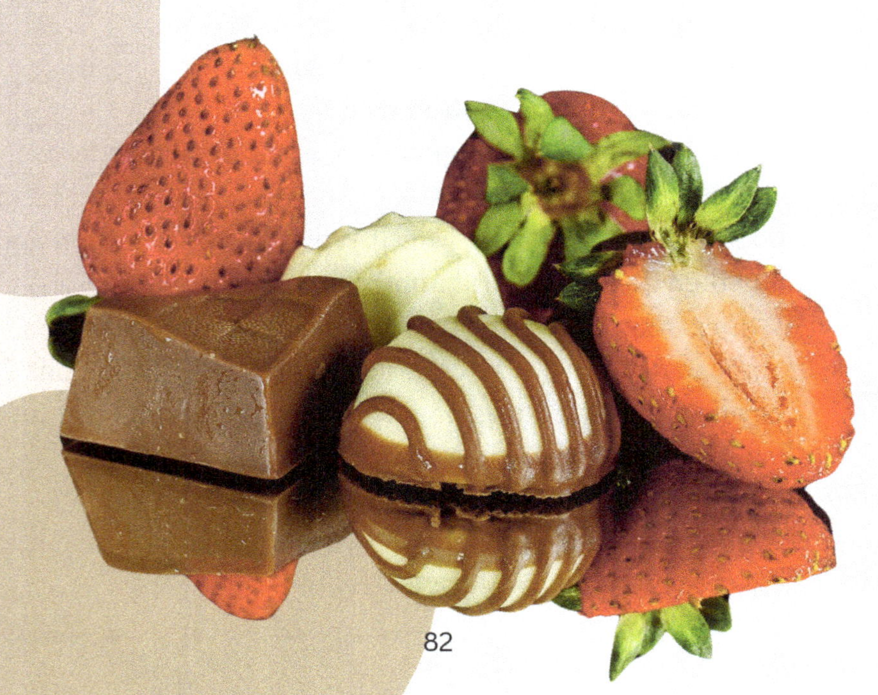

Chocolate is a common treat for humans, but it can be highly toxic to cats. Chocolate toxicity is less common in cats than in dogs, as cats are less likely to ingest chocolate; however, ingestion can still result in serious clinical signs. Cats metabolize these substances much more slowly than humans, making even small amounts of chocolate potentially dangerous.

Toxicity Level of Common Chocolate Types:

MOST to LEAST

- **White Chocolate**: Least toxic
- **Milk Chocolate:** Moderate risk, which can be a concern depending on amount ingested. Typically, toxicities are seen around 0.28 ounces per pound.
- **Dark Chocolate:** Higher risk with toxic doses beginning at around 0.11 ounces per pound.
- **Baker's Chocolate:** Very high risk; toxic doses can be at 0.05 ounces per pound.
- **Cocoa Powder**: Highest toxicity, as it is most concentrated. Toxic doses may begin at approximately 0.025 ounces per pound.

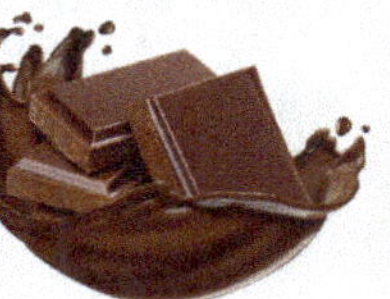

Signs of Toxicity

Severity of toxicity signs depends on the type and amount of chocolate ingested. Clinical signs are often seen within 6–12 hours of ingestion but may be delayed in some cases.

- Vomiting: This is often one of the first signs seen with toxicity.
- Diarrhea: This often accompanies vomiting and can lead to dehydration.
- Hyperactivity/Agitation: This is commonly seen as the nervous system becomes stimulated.
- Rapid Breathing: This may occur with agitation, stimulation, or overheating.
- Increased Heart Rate (Tachycardia): Elevated heart rate and abnormal rhythms can occur, leading to further complications.
- Seizures: In severe cases, neurological symptoms may arise, including seizures.

Common Interventions:

- If you suspect your cat has ingested chocolate, contact Poison Control for guidance.
- Interventions at a <u>veterinary facility</u> may include:
  - Inducing Vomiting: This may be considered depending on timeline and clinical signs.
    - Vomiting induction is much more challenging in cats than in dogs.
  - Activated Charcoal: This is rarely used in cats but may be considered.
  - Supportive Care: IV fluids and medications may be administered to manage clinical signs.

Prognosis: With appropriate and rapid response, most cats do well following chocolate ingestion.

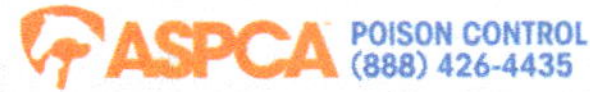

DETERGENTS

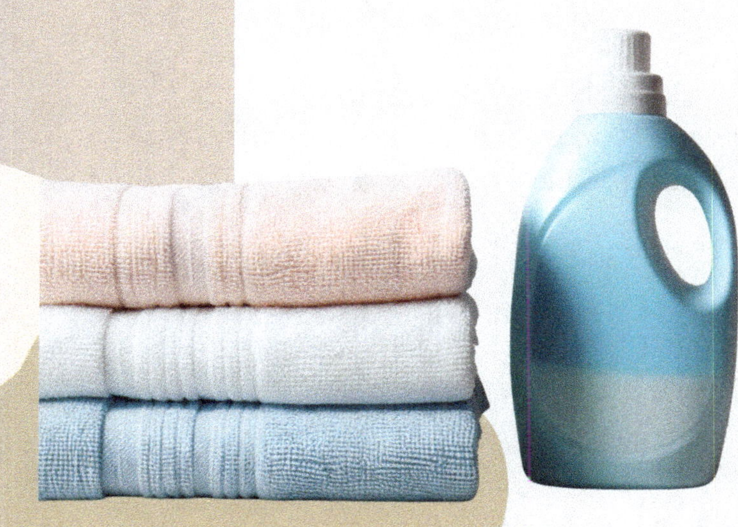

Cleaning products are a frequent source of feline exposure due to cats' grooming behavior and contact with treated surfaces. Cats may ingest residues by licking their paws or fur after walking across cleaned areas or may be exposed directly to liquids, sprays, or wipes.

Toxicity Level

Severity depends on the specific formulation, concentration, pH, and route of exposure. Many cleaning products contain a mixture of ingredients, so toxicity is not determined by product category alone. Concentrated or highly alkaline products generally pose greater risk.

Lower Risk
- Mild hand soaps and bar soaps
- Hair shampoos and conditioners
- Diluted liquid dish soap
- Low-concentration laundry detergents

Moderate Risk
- Concentrated liquid laundry detergent
- Laundry detergent pods (highly concentrated)
- Alkaline cleaning products (risk varies with concentration)

Highest Risk
- Cationic cleaning products (especially concentrated disinfectants)
- Fabric softeners
- Dishwater detergents
- Sanitizers
- Germicidal or antibacterial cleaners

Signs of Toxicity

- Clinical signs vary depending on the type of detergent, concentration, pH, and route of exposure.
- Mild exposure:
  - Drooling/ lip smacking
  - Vomiting
  - Oral irritation
- More severe exposure:
  - Difficulty swallowing
  - Coughing/ gagging
  - Profound pain
  - Ulceration of the mouth or gastrointestinal tract
  - Breathing difficulty
  - Shock (in very severe cases)

Common Interventions

- Contact Poison Control for guidance with any exposure.
- At-home monitoring may be recommended and may include:
  - Rinsing the mouth or washing the fur
  - Bread or dry food for diluted or non-corrosive detergents
  - Milk, if advised, for some corrosive materials
    - NOTE: Do not give anything by mouth if the cat is in pain, vomiting, struggling, or not alert. Only offer food or liquids if willingly accepted.
- If a veterinary visit is recommended, common interventions may include:
  - IV fluids as needed for dehydration
  - Supportive Care: treatment for nausea, pain, and ulceration
  - Hospitalization may be needed with breathing concerns.

Prognosis: With prompt decontamination and supportive care, the prognosis is generally good. Prognosis becomes more guarded with caustic products, significant oral injury, or aspiration.

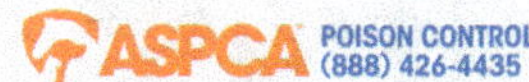

IBUPROFEN

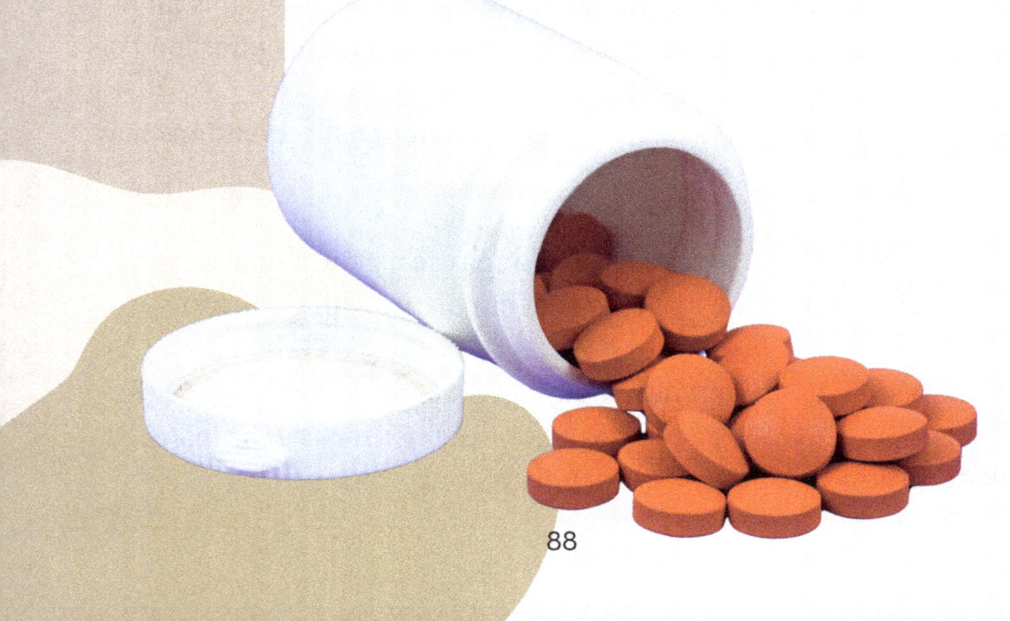

Ibuprofen is a common non-steroidal anti-inflammatory drug (NSAID) used by humans to relieve pain and inflammation and is commonly found in products such as Advil and Motrin. It is extremely dangerous to cats. Accidental exposure often occurs when pills are dropped, improperly stored, or given by well-meaning owners.

In cats, the toxic agent is Ibuprofen itself. Cats have limited pathways for drug metabolism; NSAIDs have a very narrow margin of safety and can cause gastrointestinal ulceration and kidney injury.

Toxicity Level

- Ingestion is never considered safe in cats!
- Moderate GI signs can be seen at any dose.
- Severe Gastrointestinal (GI) signs and ulcerations may be seen with ingestion of as little as 5mg/kg.
- Kidney failure may be seen at <20 mg/kg.
- Neurological effects are also possible at doses of about 200mg/kg.

Some animals will be more predisposed to the more serious side effects of an overdose.

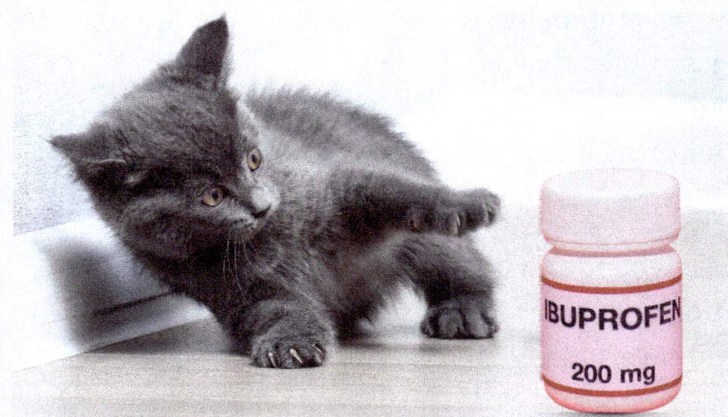

These include very small animals, older animals, or those with pre-existing kidney or liver diseases.

Signs of Toxicity

Signs are variable based on the amount of Ibuprofen ingested:
- Gastrointestinal (GI) signs:
    - Vomiting
    - Diarrhea
    - Stomach pain or discomfort
    - Black, tarry stools
- Kidney problems:
    - Increased thirst and urination
    - Lethargy
    - Kidney failure
- Nervous system signs:
    - Uncoordinated movements
    - Seizures
    - Coma (at very large doses)

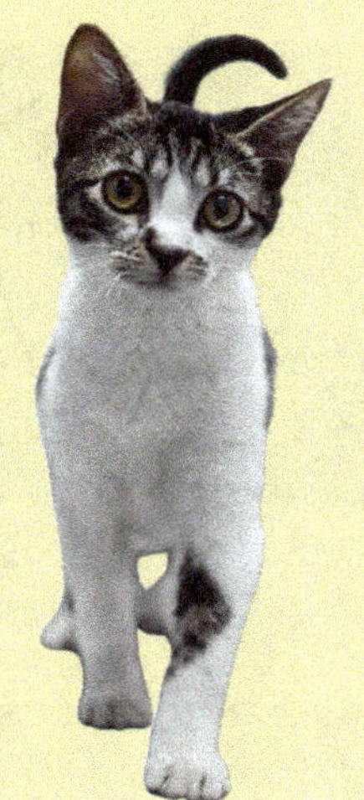

Common Interventions

- Poison Control should be contacted immediately. Veterinary care will most likely be recommended.
- At the veterinary facility, common interventions may include:
    - Inducing Vomiting - depending on the timeline
    - Administering activated charcoal
    - Baseline blood work - especially to assess kidney values
    - IV Fluids and symptomatic care - including medications to protect the gastrointestinal tract
    - Hospitalization - often for at least 48 hours
    - Ongoing monitoring and repeated blood work

Prognosis: Prognosis depends on dose and timing of treatment. With early intervention, outcomes may be fair to good; prognosis worsens with delayed care, kidney injury, or neurologic signs.

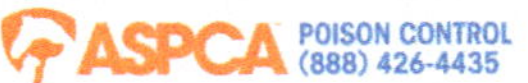

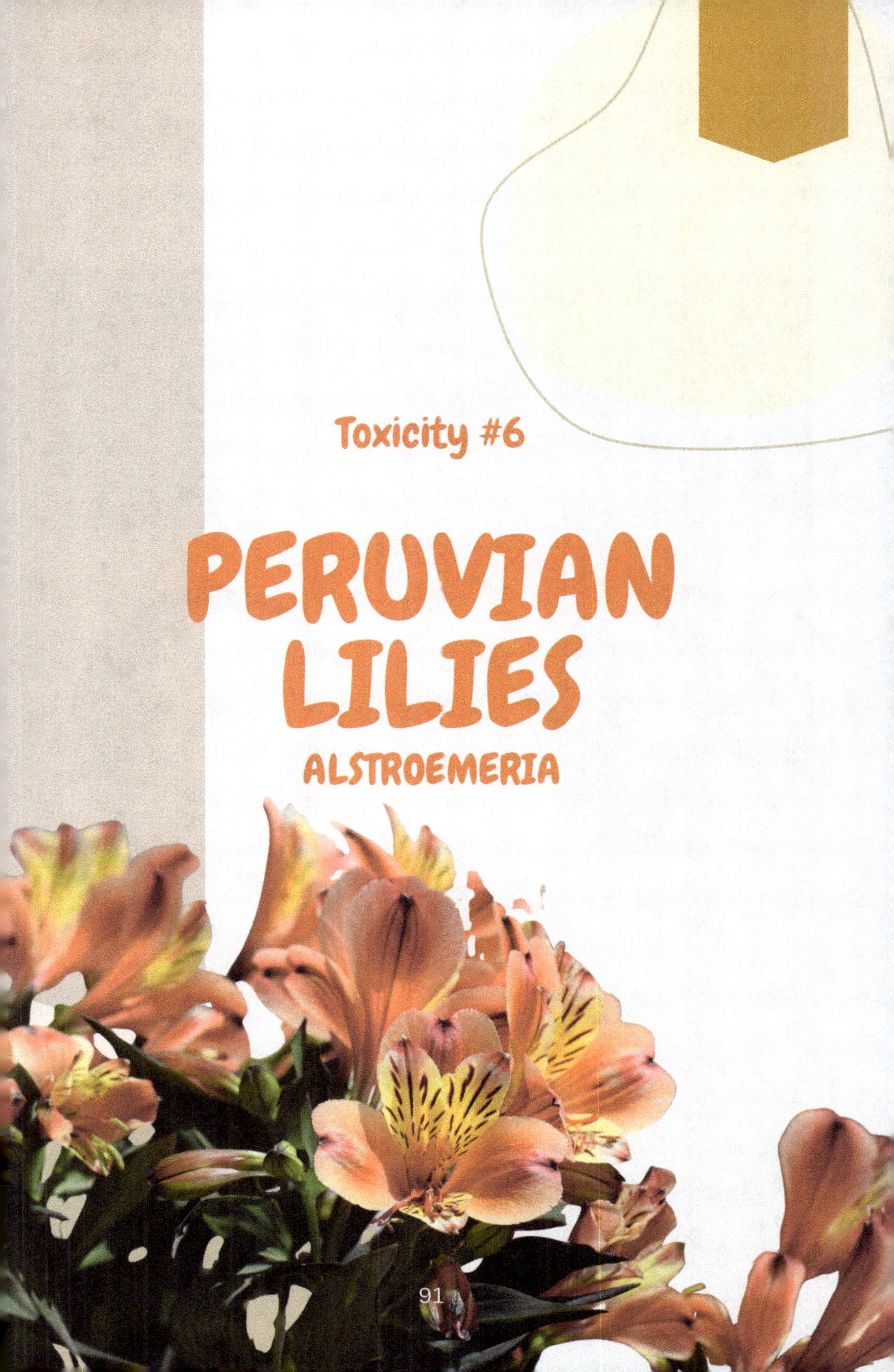

Toxicity #6

PERUVIAN LILIES

ALSTROEMERIA

Peruvian lilies are commonly mistaken for true lilies, which are well known for causing kidney failure in cats (See Toxicity #1). Unlike true lilies, Peruvian lilies do not cause kidney damage. However, ingestion can still irritate the gastrointestinal tract and lead to mild, self-limiting symptoms in some cats.

Peruvian lilies contain mild gastrointestinal irritants rather than the nephrotoxic (kidney toxic) compounds found in true lilies (such as Easter or Asiatic lilies). The exact irritating compounds are not fully characterized, but exposure primarily affects the digestive tract rather than internal organs.

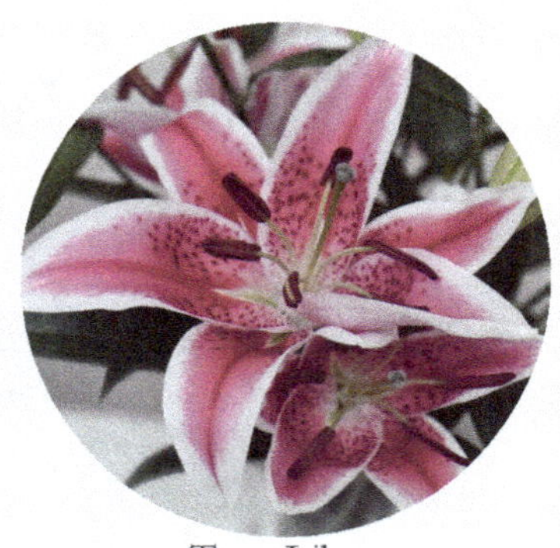

True Lily
Lilium orientalis

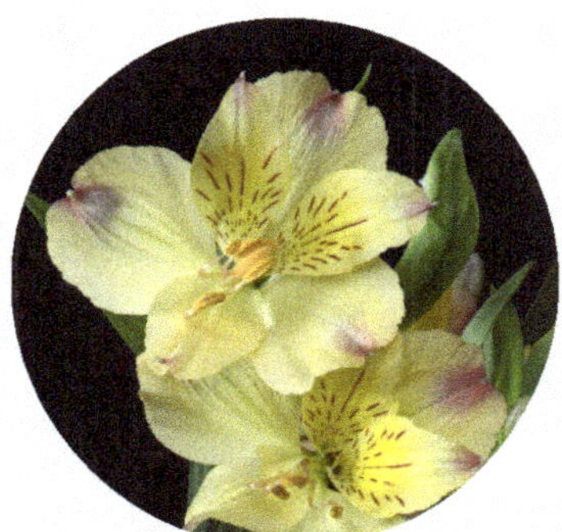

Peruvian Lily
Alstroemeria

Toxicity Level:

Toxicity level is low. This plant is not considered toxic, though exposure may cause mild gastrointestinal signs.

Signs of Toxicity

- Vomiting or diarrhea
- Mild drooling
- Decreased appetite

Signs are typically mild and self-limiting and do not usually require veterinary care.

- Contact Poison Control: Consultation with a veterinary poison service is recommended for individualized guidance.
- Emergency veterinary care is not generally recommended but may be advised depending on circumstances.
  - Cats who have pre-existing gastrointestinal upset may ingest plants as a result of nausea. As such, Poison Control may recommend a veterinary evaluation for underlying causes of nausea.
- Veterinary care may include:
  - Supportive care with supplemental fluids and anti-nausea medications.
  - Testing to assess for other underlying causes of nausea.

Prognosis: The prognosis is excellent. Clinical signs are typically mild and self-limiting, and long-term effects are not expected.

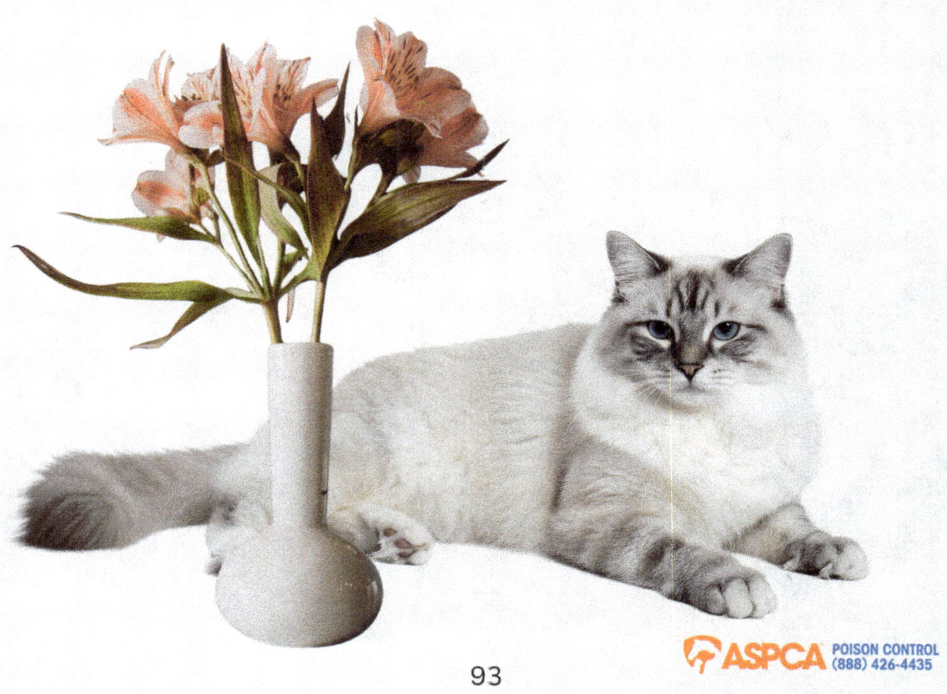

VITAMIN D

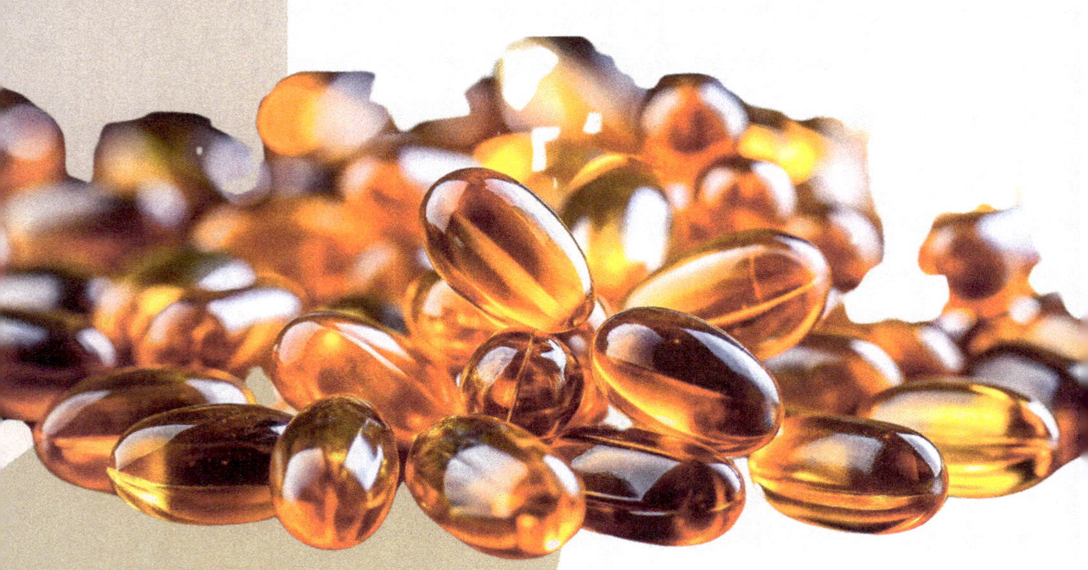

Vitamin D is essential for maintaining healthy bones and overall wellness in cats. However, excessive ingestion can lead to toxicity and serious health issues. Exposure most commonly occurs through accidental ingestion of Vitamin D supplements or cholecalciferol-containing rat bait (Vitamin D_3).

Vitamin D promotes the absorption of calcium and phosphorus in the intestines. When ingested in excessive amounts, it can cause dangerously high blood levels of calcium (hypercalcemia) and phosphorus (hyperphosphatemia), leading to calcium deposition in organs and tissues. Kidney failure may occur.

Toxicity Level

Vitamin D toxicity is dose dependent. The risk varies based on the product type and concentration. Rodenticide baits are typically far more concentrated than dietary supplements and carry a higher risk of severe poisoning.

Even small amounts relative to body weight can result in significant toxicity in cats. Ingestion of approximately 0.1 mg/kg of cholecalciferol has been associated with severe, potentially life-threatening effects, particularly with highly concentrated products. Lower-concentration supplement exposures may pose less risk depending on the calculated dose.

Note: Secondary exposure may occur in outdoor cats that consume rodents exposed to cholecalciferol rat or mouse bait. While the risk is lower than with direct ingestion, cumulative exposure over time may still result in toxicity due to the compound's long half-life.

Signs of Toxicity

Clinical signs may take several hours to a few days to appear. Signs may include:

- Early Symptoms (24-48 hours post-ingestion):
  - Vomiting
  - Loss of appetite
  - Increased thirst and urination
- Progressive Symptoms (3-7 days post-ingestion):
  - Lethargy
  - Constipation
  - Abdominal Pain
  - Muscle Tremors or Weakness
  - Kidney Failure

Common Interventions

- Contact Animal Poison Control immediately if exposure is known or suspected.
- Emergency veterinary care is often required.
- Treatment may include:
  - Inducing vomiting - depending on the timeline
  - Activated Charcoal
  - IV Fluids
  - Blood work monitoring - especially calcium, phosphorus, and kidney values. Often repeated for numerous days.
  - Medications: Cholestyramine may be used to reduce absorption by binding cholecalciferol in the intestines.
- Hospitalization needs vary based on the amount ingested and baseline blood work. Some animals may be managed on an outpatient basis with daily repeat blood work.

Prognosis: Early intervention and treatment offer the best chance for recovery. Delayed care or kidney damage significantly worsens the outcome.

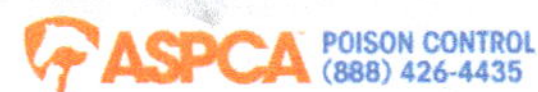

ESSENTIAL OILS

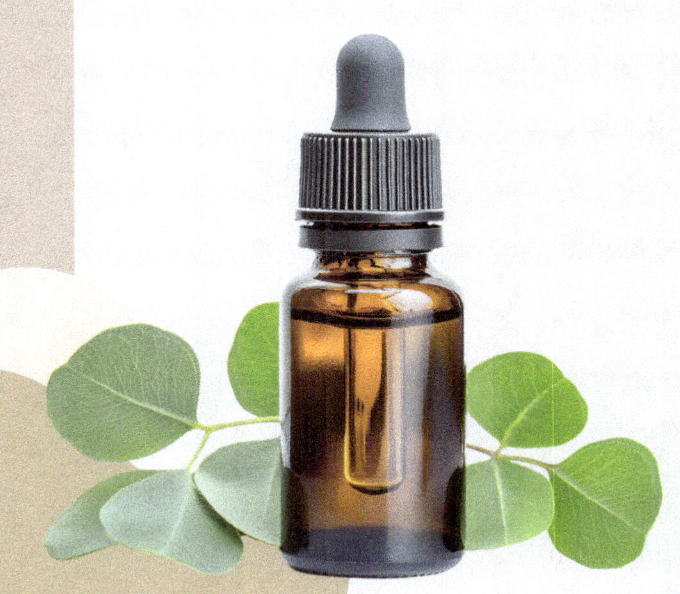

Cats are particularly sensitive to essential oils because their livers may not metabolize many of these compounds efficiently. Exposure can occur through direct contact or ingestion, as well as through inhalation from diffusers or topical products, or through grooming oil-contaminated fur or surfaces, which can lead to unintended absorption over time.

Toxin: Variable

Essential oils contain a variety of volatile organic compounds that can affect multiple body systems in cats. Depending on the specific oil and dose, these compounds may impact the liver, nervous system, and respiratory tract. Cats are especially vulnerable due to limited metabolic pathways for processing certain plant-derived chemicals, allowing these compounds to accumulate in the body.

Toxicity Level

Toxicity depends on the type of essential oil, concentration, amount and duration of exposure, and route of exposure (inhalation> ingestion> skin contact). Highly concentrated oils and repeated or prolonged exposure increase the risk of toxicity.

*NOTE: essential oils should never be used on cats without consulting a veterinarian!

Examples of common essential oils that have the potential to cause toxicity in cats

- Citronella
- Citrus
- Clove oil
- Eucalyptus
- Hyssop
- Melaleuca oil/ Tea Tree
- Pennyroyal oil
- Peppermint
- Pine
- Wintergreen

Clinical signs vary based on the type of essential oil, concentration, route, and duration of exposure. Common signs include:

- Gastrointestinal:
  - Vomiting or drooling
  - Disinterest in food
- Neurologic:
  - Weakness
  - Ataxia or instability
  - Tremors
- Respiratory: (often with aerosolized exposure)
  - Coughing
  - Wheezing
  - Trouble breathing

Common Interventions

- Contact Poison Control for guidance.
  - Immediate removal of exposure source is required.
  - Bathing the cat may be recommended.
- If a veterinary visit is recommended, common interventions may include:
  - IV fluids
  - Supportive care with management of GI signs, tremor treatment, and oxygen support.
  - Potential blood work and electrolyte monitoring
  - Hospitalization, if indicated

Prognosis: With prompt removal of exposure and appropriate care, the prognosis is generally good. Prognosis worsens with delayed treatment or severe neurologic or respiratory signs.

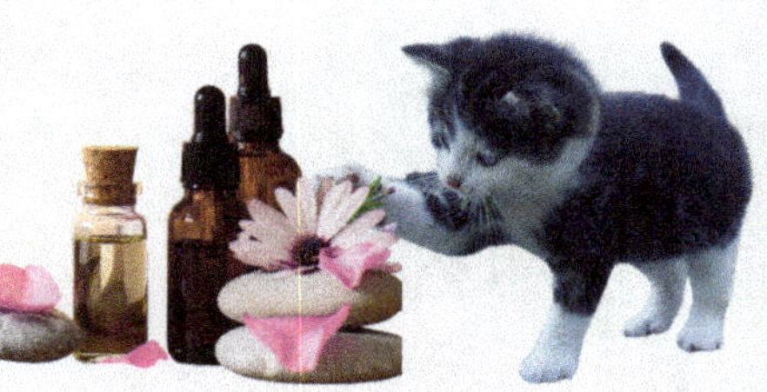

GRAPES/ RAISINS

While grapes and raisins are toxic to dogs, significant toxicity appears to be rare in cats. The specific toxic agent is not fully understood but is thought to involve tartaric acid. Although isolated cases of renal injury have been reported in cats following exposure, documented cases are uncommon.

The exact toxic agent in grapes and raisins is not fully understood. Tartaric acid and potassium bitartrate have been implicated as possible contributors, though other compounds may also play a role.

Toxicity Level

The toxic dose in cats is unknown. Reports of clinically significant toxicity in cats are rare, and there are insufficient data to establish a confirmed toxic dose. Extrapolation from canine data is not considered reliable.

There are no reported cases of toxicosis associated with ingestion of grape juice or grape jelly.

Signs of Toxicity

Clinically significant toxicity in cats appears to be rare. If signs occur, they may include:

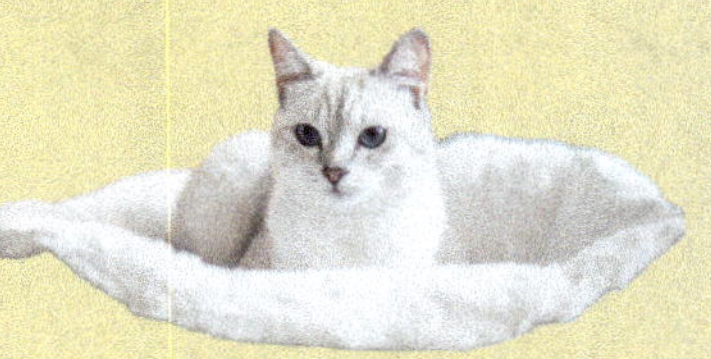

- **Initial Signs (within a few hours):**
    - Vomiting
    - Diarrhea
    - Lethargy
    - Loss of appetite

    Note: Delayed signs may be seen in the absence of early signs.
- **Delayed Signs (within 24 to 72 hours) - possible, though unlikely:**
    - Increased thirst and urination
    - Abdominal pain
    - Kidney failure

Common Interventions

- Contact Poison Control with any ingestion and discuss further recommendations. A veterinary visit may be advised.
- Common interventions at a veterinary facility may include:
  - Inducing vomiting - to attempt to recover grapes/raisins
  - Medications - to control vomiting and settle the stomach
  - IV Fluids - typically administered for at least 48 hours
  - Repeat blood work - to monitor kidney function; typically for at least 72 hours

Prognosis: With rapid intervention and no signs of kidney failure within 72 hours of ingestion, the prognosis is very good, and long-term complications are unlikely. Prognosis becomes less favorable if kidney failure does occur.

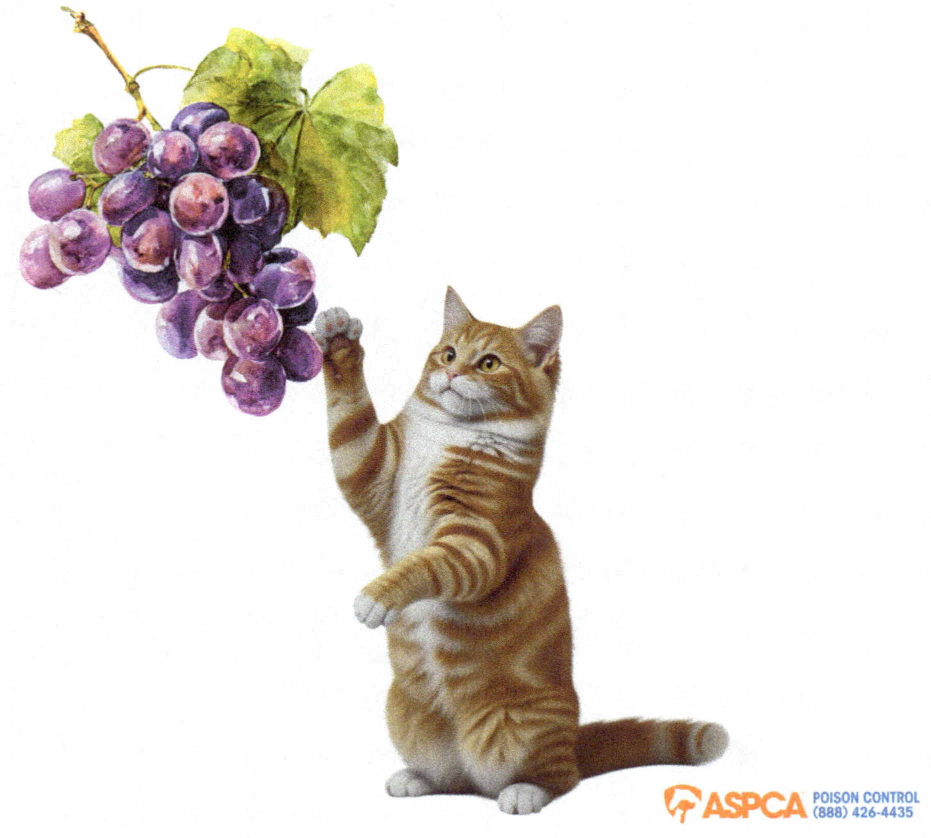

CARPROFEN

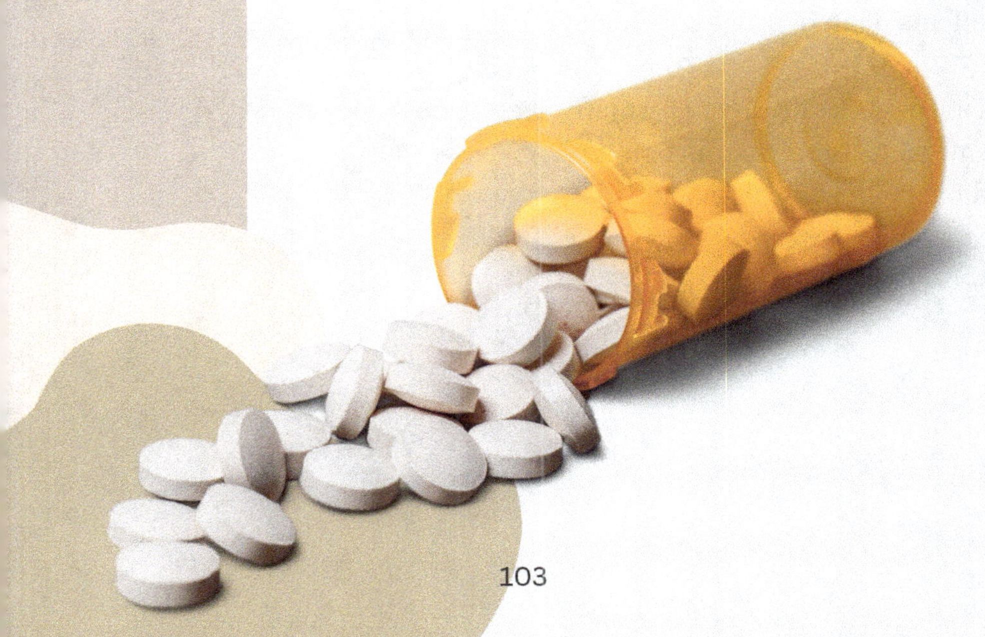

Carprofen is a non-steroidal anti-inflammatory drug (NSAID) that is commonly prescribed for dogs to relieve pain and inflammation. While carprofen is safe for dogs at prescribed dosages, it can be toxic to cats due to their limited ability to metabolize these medications through the liver.

Toxicity Level

- Ingestion is never considered safe in cats!
- Moderate gastrointestinal signs can be seen at any dose.
- Severe gastrointestinal ulceration has been reported with ingestion of as little as ~2.9 mg/kg.
- Kidney failure may occur at doses of ~8 mg/kg.
- Neurologic effects are possible at very high doses (reported around ~200 mg/kg).

Some animals will be more predisposed to the more serious side effects of an overdose.

These include very small animals, older animals, or those with pre-existing kidney or liver diseases.

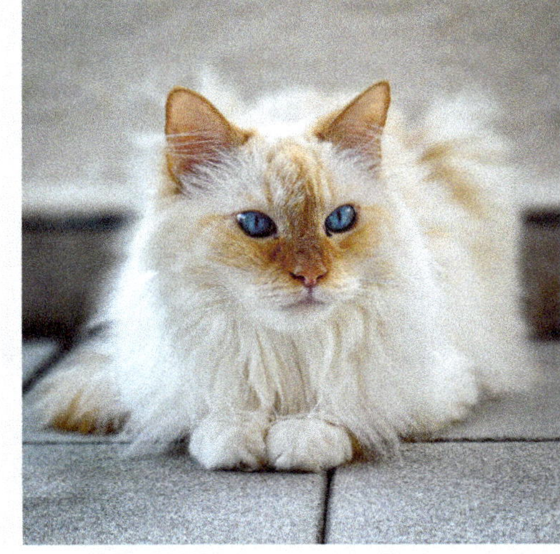

Clinical signs vary based on the amount of carprofen ingested:
- Gastrointestinal (GI) signs:
  - Vomiting
  - Diarrhea
  - Stomach pain or discomfort
  - Black, tarry stools
- Kidney problems:
  - Increased thirst and urination
  - Lethargy
  - Kidney failure
- Nervous system signs (possible with very high exposure):
  - Uncoordinated movements
  - Seizures

Common Interventions

- Animal Poison Control should be contacted immediately. Veterinary care will most likely be recommended.
- At the veterinary facility, common interventions may include:
  - Inducing vomiting - depending on the timeline
  - Administering activated charcoal
  - Baseline blood work - especially to assess kidney values
  - IV fluids and supportive care - including medications to protect the gastrointestinal tract
  - Hospitalization - often for at least 48 - 72hours
  - Ongoing monitoring and repeated blood work

Prognosis: Prognosis depends on the dose ingested and how quickly treatment is started. With early intervention, outcomes may be fair to good; prognosis worsens with delayed care, kidney injury, or severe gastrointestinal ulceration.

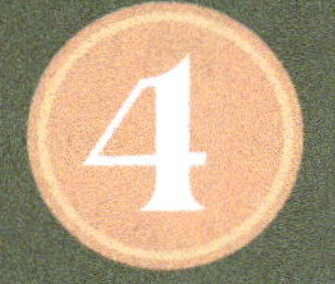

HOW TO RECOGNIZE AN EMERGENCY

(COMMON SIGNS THAT OFTEN INDICATE AN EMERGENCY)

Determining whether your cat's signs are serious enough to warrant an emergency visit can be challenging. A helpful rule of thumb is this: If your cat is behaving unusually or showing signs of distress, it's wise to err on the side of caution. Contact your veterinarian or an emergency clinic for guidance.

Cats are especially skilled at **hiding illness and pain**. Subtle changes in behavior, appetite, posture, or routine may be the only outward clues that something is wrong. Because of this, signs that seem mild can sometimes reflect serious underlying conditions.

While minor issues like itchy skin, a mildly upset stomach, or slight limping may not require urgent care, there are specific situations that demand immediate action. Below is a list of common signs that should prompt a response from you. Sometimes this means calling your veterinarian for advice. Other times, immediate evaluation by an urgent care or emergency (ER) veterinarian is necessary.

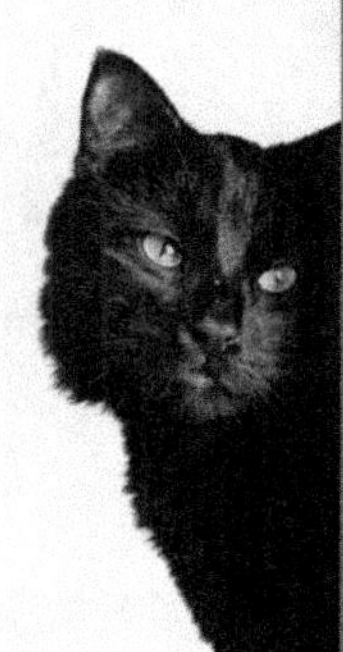

Chapter Highlights

Critical Signs that Should Not be Ignored:

1. Difficulty Breathing
2. Urinary Issues
3. Collapse or Weakness
4. Trauma
5. Bleeding
6. Severe Vomiting or Diarrhea
7. Severe Pain or Difficulty Moving
8. Sudden Lethargy or Behavior Change
9. Tremors or Seizures
10. Acute Blindness

OVERVIEW

- Panting
- Respiratory Effort
- Respiratory Rate
- Accompanying Signs of Concern

True Emergency!

DIFFICULTY BREATHING

SKILLS TOOLKIT

- Resting Respiratory Rate

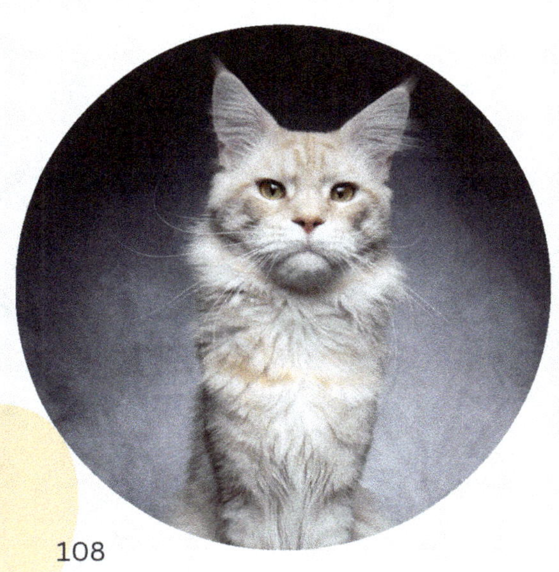

Breathing concerns can be difficult to interpret, especially in cats. Because cats are skilled at hiding illness and pain, changes in breathing may be subtle or easy to miss.

Respiratory problems can worsen quickly, so it is important to recognize abnormal signs and seek veterinary guidance promptly when concerns arise. If you are ever unsure or feel that something is not right, trust your instincts and seek veterinary care rather than delaying.

Panting

Unlike dogs, panting is not a normal behavior in cats. Open-mouth breathing, rapid breathing, or panting in a cat is often a sign of significant respiratory distress, pain, overheating, or underlying disease. If your cat is panting or breathing with an open mouth, this should be treated as an emergency and prompt veterinary evaluation is recommended.

Respiratory Effort

Changes in breathing effort can be an important sign of respiratory distress in cats. Normal feline breathing is quiet and subtle, with minimal visible movement.

Abdominal contractions: Abdominal contractions refer to exaggerated movement of the belly during breathing. If your cat's abdomen is pulling in and out forcefully with each breath, this may indicate that breathing requires increased effort.

If you notice pronounced abdominal movement, visible effort when breathing, or a "heaving" motion of the belly, your cat may be struggling to breathe. This is a serious concern and requires emergency assessment.

Difficulty breathing is medically referred to as <u>dyspnea.</u>

Respiratory Rate

Knowing your cat's normal respiratory rate can help you recognize early signs of breathing trouble.

Resting Respiratory Rate (RRR): Respiratory rate should always be assessed while your cat is calm and resting, not after activity or during stressful situations.

- To determine the RRR, count the number of times their chest rises and falls in one minute. You can count for six seconds and multiply by ten to find the breaths per minute.
- Typically, a healthy cat's respiratory rate is <u>fewer than 30 breaths per minute</u>.
- Keep in mind that individual rates can vary. If you notice a consistent increase in your cat's breathing rate, it could be a cause for concern.
- Do NOT count panting as an elevated respiratory rate. Panting or open-mouth breathing is not normal in cats and is concerning.

A rapid respiratory rate is known as <u>tachypnea.</u>

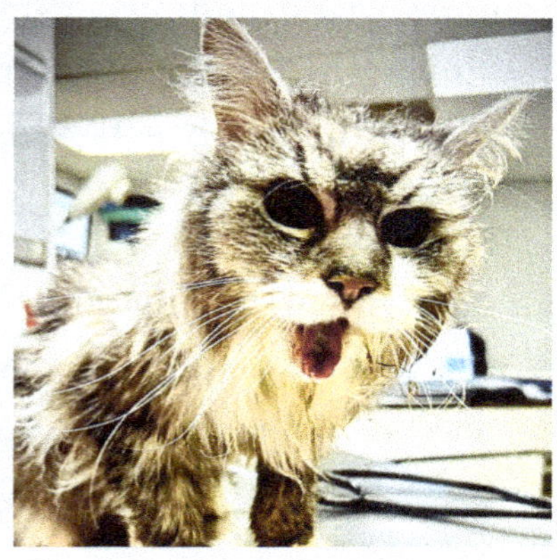

Figure 4.1: Cats should never breathe with their mouths open. Unlike dogs, open-mouth breathing in cats, with or without discoloration of the tongue or gums (cyanosis), is a medical emergency.

Photo credit: Dr. A Gavin Smith

Signs that Accompany Respiratory Distress

When a cat is in respiratory distress, you may notice several accompanying changes in addition to an increased respiratory rate or effort:

- **General Discomfort**: Signs may include restlessness, agitation, hiding, reluctance to move, or an inability to get comfortable.
- **Sleep Changes**: Cats may have difficulty resting comfortably, may avoid lying down, or may remain upright for extended periods.
- **Eating Changes:** Difficulty breathing can lead to decreased appetite or refusal of food as the cat focuses its energy on breathing.
- **Neck Extension:** In severe cases, cats may extend their neck or hold their head and body in an abnormal position to help improve airflow.
- **Abnormal Respiratory Sounds:** Breathing may sound noisy, raspy, or congested. While coughing is less common in cats than dogs, any unusual breathing sounds can indicate an underlying problem.
- **Gum Color Changes:** In severe cases, decreased oxygen delivery or poor circulation can cause the gums to appear pale or bluish (cyanosis).

If you observe any of these signs, it is important to seek emergency veterinary care.

SUMMARY:

Respiratory distress requires prompt attention. Changes in breathing, behavior, or posture may be early warning signs. If breathing seems abnormal, seek veterinary care right away.

OVERVIEW

- Signs
- Potential Causes
- When to Seek Veterinary Care

SKILLS TOOLKIT

- How to Palpate a Bladder

Possible Emergency

URINARY ISSUES

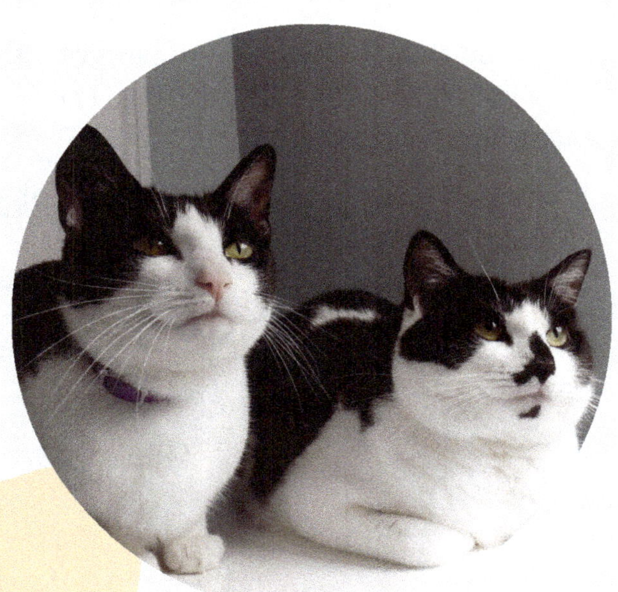

Urinary emergencies are common in cats and can become serious very quickly. While severe urinary complications can occur in any cat, male cats are far more likely to develop life-threatening urinary obstructions. Cats often show subtle or vague signs of urinary discomfort and delays in seeking care can lead to significant complications. Because cats may hide pain or illness, any change in urination or litter box habits should be taken seriously.

Some urinary concerns may warrant monitoring or veterinary advice, while others require immediate emergency care. If you are ever unsure whether a urinary change is serious, trust your instincts and seek veterinary guidance rather than waiting.

Signs of a Urinary Emergency

Urinary emergencies often present with a combination of litter box changes, discomfort, and behavior changes. The following signs should raise concern:

- **Straining or repeated attempts to urinate,** especially with little or no urine produced
- **Vocalizing or signs of pain** during or after litter box use
- **Frequent litter box visits** or prolonged time in the box
- **Blood-tinged** urine
- **Urinating outside the litter box**
- **Lethargy, vomiting, or worsening weakness**

If these signs are present, veterinary evaluation is recommended. If your cat appears unable to urinate, this is an emergency.

Inability to Urinate

A cat that is unable to pass urine is experiencing a medical emergency.

If your cat is repeatedly straining in the litter box and producing little to no urine, this should be treated as an emergency situation. Urinary obstruction can rapidly lead to serious complications and is most commonly seen in male cats, though it can occur in any cat.

If you suspect your cat is unable to urinate, do not wait to see if the signs improve. Seek emergency veterinary care immediately.

How to Palpate the Bladder at Home

Becoming familiar with how your cat's bladder feels, especially in male cats, can be a useful tool when there are urinary concerns.

Please note that not all cats will tolerate bladder palpation, and this should only be attempted if your cat is calm and comfortable with handling.

Palpation technique:
- Allow your cat to remain standing on a stable surface.
- Using one hand, gently cup the lower abdomen from underneath, just in front of the hind legs *(See Figure 4.3)*.
- With your hand cupped, scoop backward toward the tail while lightly lifting upward, using minimal pressure.
- Observe both what you feel and how your cat responds.

Figure 4.2: Diagram showing the bladder location

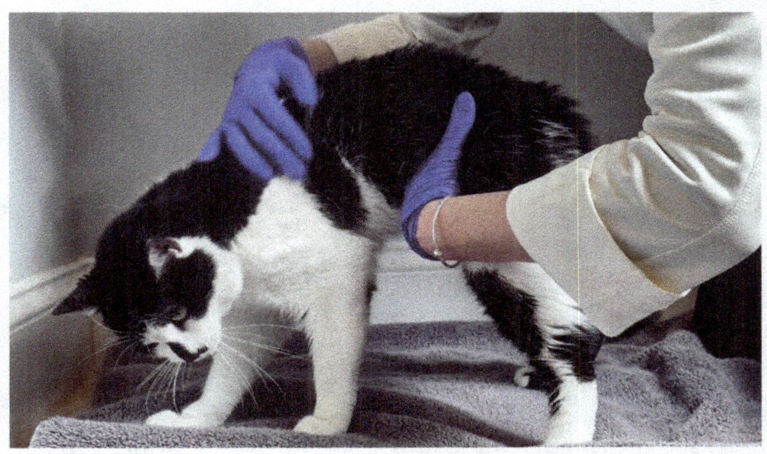

Figure 4.3: An image depicting accurate positioning for a cat during urinary bladder palpation

Photo credit: F. Ducharme

Interpretation:

Many owners will not be able to feel a normal urinary bladder, as it is often small and subtle, especially if the bladder has recently been emptied. A bladder that is abnormally full is more likely to feel noticeable.

In general:
- If your cat is not demonstrating signs of urinary issues, the bladder will likely be **small** and may be difficult to feel.
  - Becoming familiar with this can be helpful for comparison if concerns arise later.
- A bladder that feels **large, firm, or hard** is concerning, particularly if your cat is straining to urinate or showing other urinary signs. In this situation, veterinary evaluation should not be delayed.

When to Seek Veterinary Care

Veterinary evaluation is recommended for any cat showing changes in urination or litter box behavior, especially if signs persist or worsen.

Seek immediate emergency care if:
- Your cat is straining to urinate with little or no urine produced
- You suspect your cat is unable to urinate
- A bladder feels firm, hard, or enlarged upon gentle palpation
- Urinary signs are accompanied by lethargy, vomiting, weakness, or signs of pain

Urinary obstruction is most common in male cats, but any cat with urinary signs should be evaluated promptly.
If you are unsure whether a situation is urgent, it is always safer to seek veterinary guidance rather than wait.

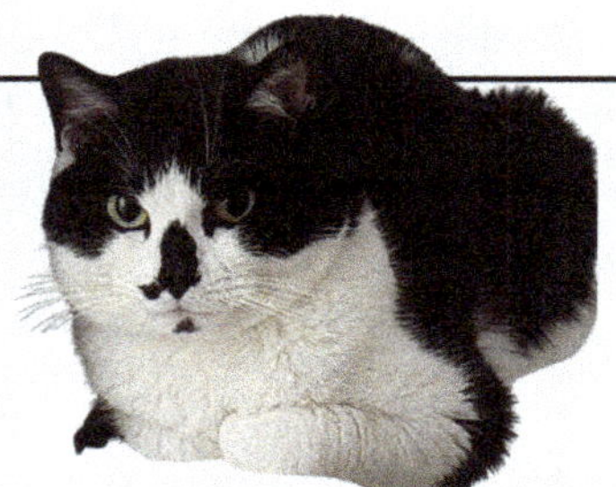

SUMMARY:

Urinary signs in cats can have many underlying causes, ranging from mild and temporary changes to life-threatening emergencies such as urinary obstruction. Because these conditions often look similar at home, it can be difficult to determine severity without veterinary evaluation. Signs such as straining to urinate, producing little to no urine, vocalizing, lethargy, or a firm, enlarged bladder warrant prompt veterinary attention. When in doubt, it is always safest to err on the side of caution and seek veterinary care.

OVERVIEW

- Signs
- Potential Causes
- When to Seek Veterinary Care

SKILLS TOOLKIT

- Collapse Response Steps

True Emergency!

COLLAPSE

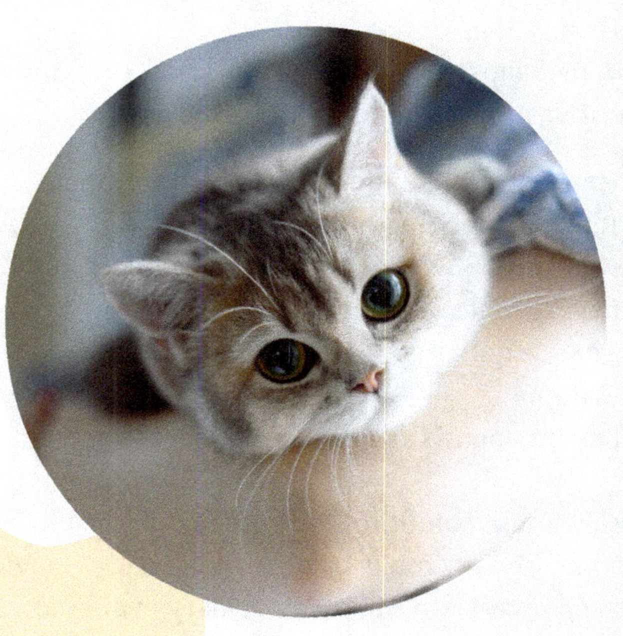

Sudden collapse or a rapid onset of severe weakness is always concerning in cats and may indicate a serious underlying problem. These changes can occur abruptly and should not be ignored.

Cats do not need to fully lose consciousness for this to be serious. Any sudden inability to stand, walk, or support normal body posture warrants concern.

Signs of Collapse/Severe Weakness

You may notice one or more of the following signs:

- Sudden inability to stand or walk normally
- Stumbling, swaying, or loss of balance
- Inability to support normal body posture
- Abrupt reluctance or inability to move
- Extreme lethargy with minimal response to surroundings
- Pale gums
- Rapid or labored breathing

Common Causes

Sudden collapse or severe weakness in cats can result from a variety of serious medical conditions, including:

- Heart disease or abnormal heart rhythms
- Internal bleeding
- Neurologic disease
- Severe metabolic disturbances
- Toxin exposure
- Trauma
- Severe anemia

Because these conditions can present with similar outward signs and may not be externally visible, it is not possible to determine the cause or severity at home. Veterinary evaluation is necessary.

What to Do if Your Cat Collapses or is Severely Weak

- **Minimize handling.** Speak to your cat and note whether they respond to your voice or movement.
- **Assess breathing.** Note rapid, labored, or abnormal breathing.
- **Check briefly for obvious injury or bleeding** if trauma is suspected.
- **Prepare for transport.** Place your cat in a carrier or secure box lined with a towel, keeping movement to a minimum.
- **Proceed to a veterinary facility**. Transport your cat in a carrier or secure box and *call ahead if possible.*

When to Seek Veterinary Care

Any episode of sudden collapse or severe weakness warrants prompt veterinary evaluation - even if your cat appears to recover quickly.

Seek emergency care if:
- Your cat suddenly cannot stand, walk, or support normal posture
- Weakness is severe, sudden, or worsening
- Episodes of collapse come and go
- Collapse or weakness is accompanied by pale gums or breathing difficulty

If you are unsure whether a change is serious, it is safest to seek veterinary care rather than wait.

SUMMARY:

Sudden collapse or severe weakness in cats can have many possible causes, some of which are life-threatening. Because it is not possible to determine the cause or severity at home, abrupt changes in strength or mobility should prompt veterinary evaluation. When in doubt, err on the side of caution and seek veterinary care.

OVERVIEW

- Minor Trauma
- Major Trauma
- When to Seek Veterinary Care

SKILLS TOOLKIT

- Trauma Response

Possible Emergency

TRAUMA
(PHYSICAL INJURY)

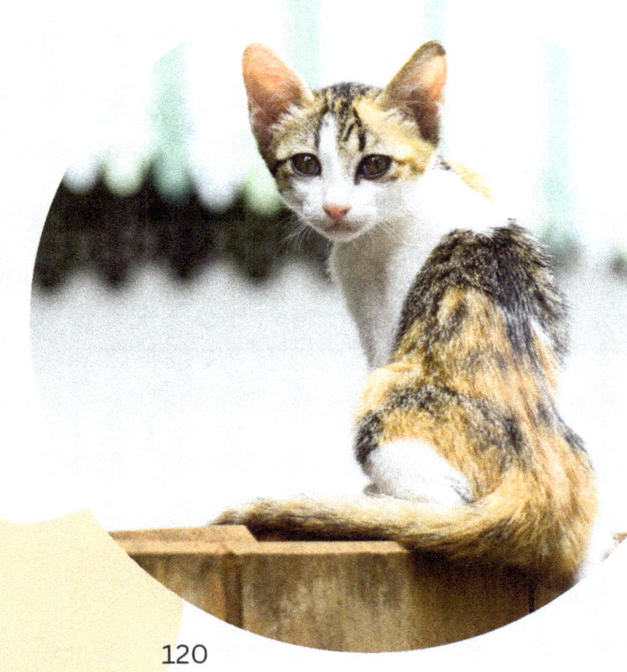

Trauma refers to physical injury caused by an accident or force and can range from mild to life-threatening. In cats, even injuries that appear minor can result in serious internal damage. Because cats often hide pain and may limit movement after an injury, trauma is not always immediately obvious.

Any known or suspected traumatic event should be taken seriously.

Types of Trauma

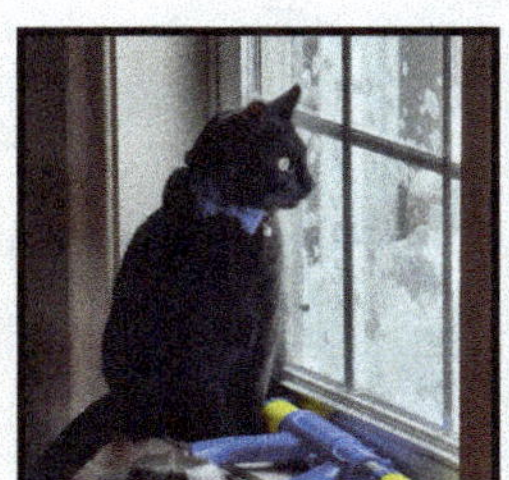

Trauma in cats may occur after:

- Falls from furniture, counters, or windows
- Falls from significant heights
- Being struck by a vehicle
- Animal bites or fights
- Being accidentally stepped on, trapped, or crushed

The severity of injury depends on both the type of trauma and your cat's response afterward, not just how dramatic the incident appeared.

Signs of Trauma

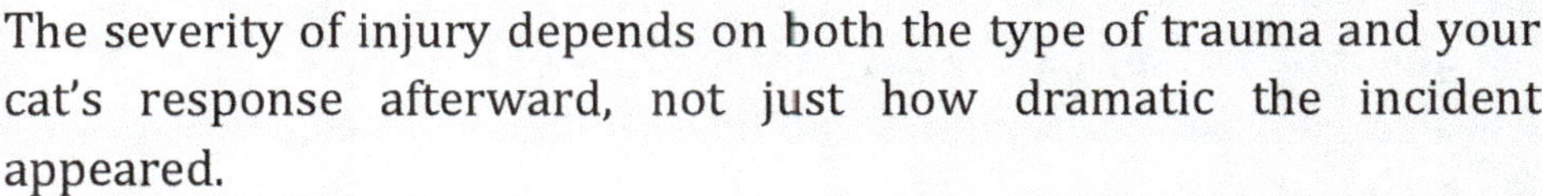

After an injury or suspected accident, watch for the following signs:

- Limping or inability to use a limb
- Difficulty standing, walking, or jumping
- Pain when touched or reluctance to move
- Hunched posture or guarding a body part
- Visible wounds, swelling, or bleeding
- Rapid or labored breathing
- Pale gums
- Sudden lethargy, weakness, or collapse
- Changes in behavior, such as hiding or decreased responsiveness

Loss of consciousness, even briefly, is always concerning.

Some injuries, including internal bleeding, fractures, or head trauma, may not be visible externally. A cat may appear quiet or withdrawn rather than overtly painful, which can delay recognition of serious injury.

Because of this, the true severity of trauma cannot be reliably determined at home.

What to Do if Your Cat Experiences Trauma

- **Minimize handling.** Allow your cat to remain as still as possible and avoid unnecessary movement.
- **Check** briefly for visible bleeding or obvious injury. Apply gentle pressure if bleeding is present.
- **Observe** your cat closely for pain, limping, weakness, breathing changes, or behavior changes.
- **Contact a veterinarian** for guidance if you are unsure whether the injury is serious or how urgently care is needed.
- **Proceed to a veterinary facility** if injuries appear significant, signs worsen, or veterinary guidance recommends evaluation.

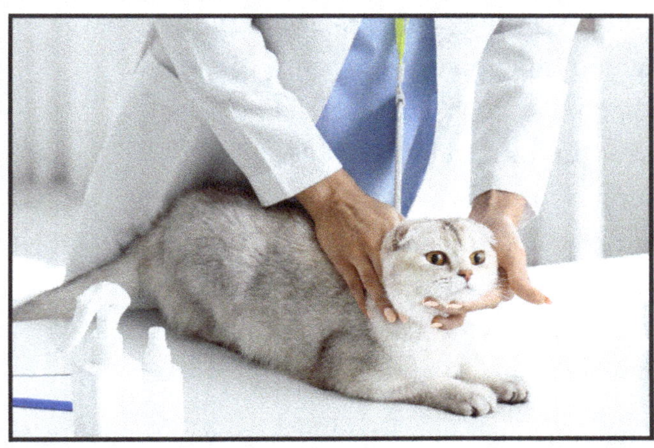

When to Seek Veterinary Care

Veterinary evaluation is recommended for any cat that has experienced trauma, even if injuries appear mild at first.

Seek urgent or emergency veterinary care if:
- Your cat is unable or unwilling to stand, walk, or use a limb
- There is ongoing or uncontrolled bleeding
- Breathing is abnormal or labored
- Your cat appears painful, weak, collapsed, or unusually quiet
- There is any loss of consciousness, even briefly

Because cats may hide pain and internal injuries are not always visible, it is safer to seek veterinary care rather than wait if concerning signs are present.

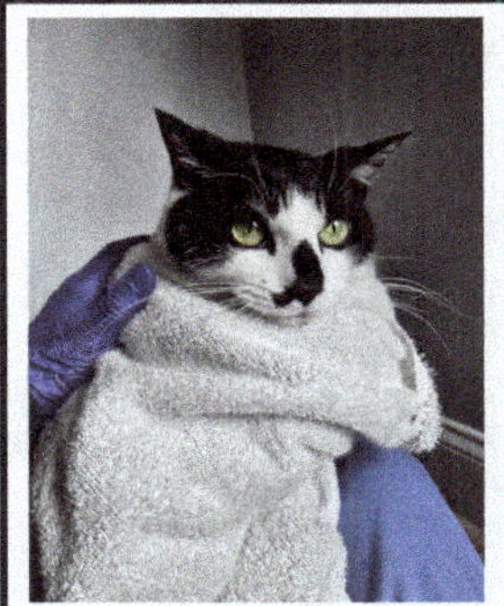

Use caution when moving a cat after trauma. Painful cats may bite or scratch. A towel or small blanket can help with safe handling.

Photo credit: R. Ducharme

SUMMARY:

Trauma in cats can range from mild to life-threatening, and the severity of injury is not always immediately apparent. Because cats often hide pain and internal injuries cannot be assessed at home, even seemingly minor trauma should be monitored closely. If concerning signs develop or if you are unsure how serious an injury may be, veterinary evaluation is recommended. When in doubt, err on the side of caution and seek professional care.

OVERVIEW

- External Bleeding
- Internal Bleeding
- Signs of Significant Blood Loss
- When to Seek Veterinary Care

SKILLS TOOLKIT

- Managing Simple External Bleeding

Possible Emergency

BLEEDING

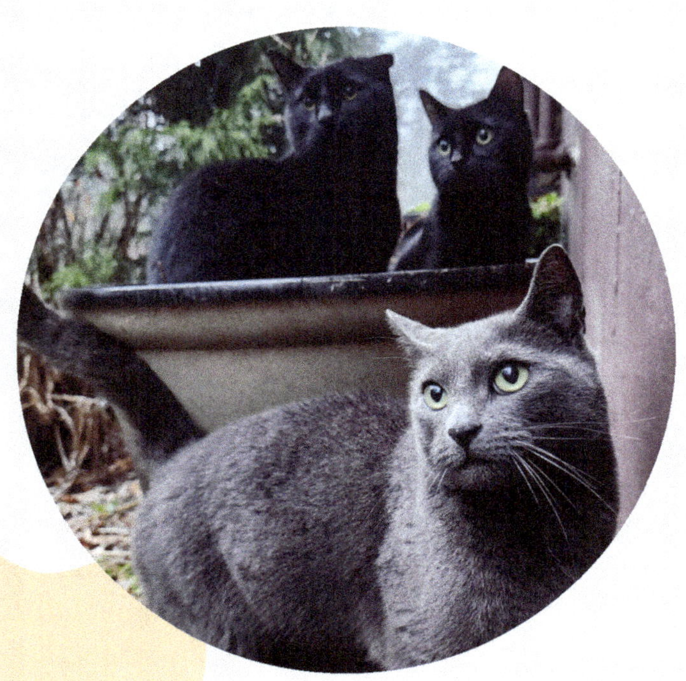

Bleeding in cats can be external or internal and may range from minor to life-threatening. While simple external bleeding can sometimes be managed at home with first aid, internal bleeding always requires veterinary care. Because cats may hide pain and blood loss, bleeding should be taken seriously.

Recognizing and Managing External and Internal Bleeding

EXTERNAL Bleeding

External bleeding is bleeding you can see, such as from a wound, toenail, or the mouth or nose. Minor external bleeding can sometimes be controlled with basic first aid.

How to Manage External Bleeding

For minor wounds or toenail injuries:
- <u>Apply Pressure:</u> Firm, consistent pressure is key to stopping the bleeding. Resist the urge to check too soon. Keep applying pressure for at least five minutes to allow a clot to form.
- <u>Clotting Aids:</u>
  - For TOENAILS only: If bleeding persists, you can use baking soda, cornstarch, or baking powder to help form a clot.
- Note: Depending on the cause of the bleeding, veterinary care may still be needed even if bleeding has stopped.
  - Wounds can easily become infected and often require veterinary evaluation.

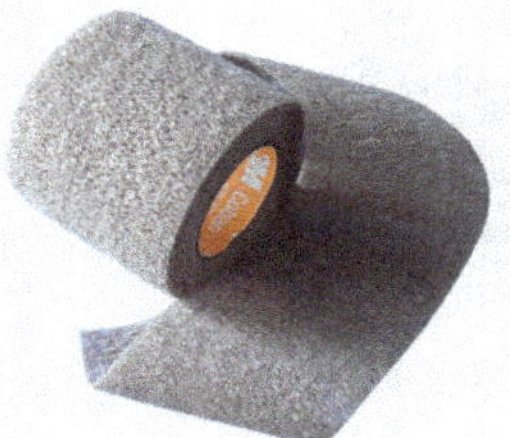

Internal bleeding cannot be seen and may occur after trauma, toxin exposure (like rat bait), or due to underlying medical conditions. Since the blood isn't visible, it's important to watch for signs of blood loss or anemia.

Signs of Significant Blood Loss in Cats:

- **Pale or white gums:** This is often a sign of reduced blood in circulation.
  - While there are other causes for pale gums, those always require a veterinary assessment.
- **Weakness or lethargy:** Reduced energy, reluctance to move, or sudden quietness may occur as circulating blood volume decreases.
- **Rapid or shallow breathing:** Breathing may become faster or more effortful as the body attempts to compensate for reduced oxygen delivery.
- **Cold extremities:** Ears, paws, or limbs may feel cooler than normal due to poor circulation.
- **Behavioral changes**: Cats may become unusually quiet, withdrawn, disoriented, or less responsive than normal.
- **Dilated pupils**: Enlarged pupils may be seen in severe cases and can be associated with shock or reduced blood flow.
- **Collapse or severe weakness:** In advanced cases, significant blood loss may lead to collapse.

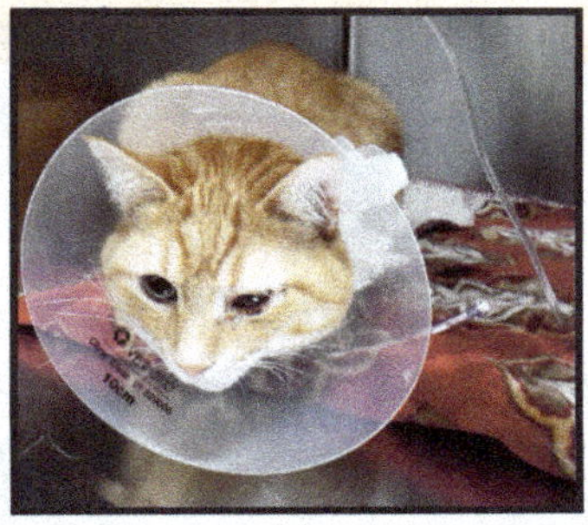

Photo credit: Dr. J Karau

Any cat with bleeding should be monitored closely, as even small amounts of blood loss can become significant. While minor external bleeding may stop with direct pressure, veterinary evaluation is recommended if bleeding continues, the wound appears deep, or the injury is painful.

Seek urgent or emergency veterinary care if:
- Bleeding does not stop after several minutes of steady pressure
- A wound is large, deep, or caused by a bite
- Your cat shows signs that may be associated with internal bleeding, such as pale gums, weakness, collapse, or breathing changes
- Bleeding is accompanied by marked lethargy or behavioral changes

Because internal bleeding cannot be seen and cats often hide signs of illness, it is safer to seek veterinary care rather than wait when bleeding is present.

SUMMARY:

Bleeding can range from minor external injuries to serious, life-threatening conditions. While simple external bleeding may be controlled with direct pressure, ongoing bleeding, deep wounds, or signs of blood loss require veterinary evaluation. Because internal bleeding cannot be assessed at home, cats showing signs of blood loss should receive prompt veterinary care. When in doubt, err on the side of caution and seek veterinary care.

OVERVIEW

- Vomiting
  - Acute vs Intermittent
- A Note About Hairballs
- Diarrhea
- Signs of Dehydration
- Accompanying Signs of Concern

SKILLS TOOLKIT

- Evaluating Dehydration
  - Gum Moisture Assessment
  - Eye Assessment
  - Skin Tenting
  - Capillary Refill Times

True Emergency!

SEVERE/PERSISTENT VOMITING/ DIARRHEA

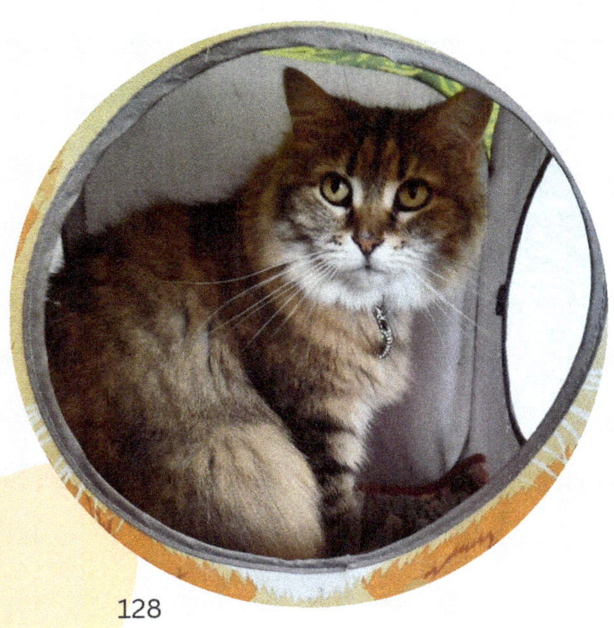

Vomiting and diarrhea are among the most common reasons cats are brought to the emergency clinic. While occasional vomiting or loose stools can occur and are often related to dietary indiscretion or mild gastrointestinal upset, persistent or severe gastrointestinal signs warrant prompt veterinary attention.

Because these issues are so common, it can be difficult for cat owners to know when to be concerned. As a general rule, if vomiting or diarrhea is persistent, worsening, or accompanied by behavior changes, lethargy, or blood, veterinary evaluation is recommended.

Persistent/ Frequent Vomiting

If your cat vomits more than two to three times within a 12-hour period, veterinary evaluation is recommended. Repeated vomiting can quickly lead to dehydration in cats and may signal a more serious underlying problem, such as gastrointestinal obstruction, toxin exposure, or systemic illness.
When assessing vomiting, it is important to consider associated behavior changes, as these can provide valuable insight into severity.

Lethargy:
- Lethargy, or unusual fatigue, is often seen in conjunction with vomiting. A lethargic cat may have reduced energy, show little interest in normal activities, disengage from family members, or hide. While some lethargy can occur naturally after vomiting, it is important to monitor your cat's behavior closely.
- Persistent lethargy, especially when combined with vomiting, may indicate dehydration, low blood pressure, low blood sugar, or an underlying systemic problem.
- If your cat remains lethargic for several hours after vomiting and does not return to normal activity, veterinary evaluation is recommended. If your cat is unwilling to move, minimally responsive, or appears profoundly unwell, this is an emergency requiring immediate veterinary care.

- A sudden refusal to eat after vomiting is not uncommon and is usually a protective response. However, this loss of appetite should not last for more than 24 hours.
- If your cat continues to show no interest in food or if there is a gradual decline in appetite over several days, this is a red flag.
- Cats that fail to eat for extended periods can rapidly develop secondary issues, such as further dehydration or nutritional deficiencies, which can complicate the situation.

What About Acute Vomiting?

If your cat vomits once or twice and is otherwise acting normally with no signs of lethargy, the situation may be less urgent.

- A crucial factor to consider with acute vomiting is whether your cat was **fasted** after the vomiting occurred. *Many pet owners, with the best intentions, offer food or water right after vomiting, thinking it will prevent dehydration. However, this can often make the situation worse.*
  - When a cat vomits, their stomach becomes inflamed. Introducing food or water (or not restricting access to them) can further irritate the stomach and lead to <u>more</u> vomiting.
    - For this reason, we recommend withholding food and water for at least 6-8 hours after the first instance of vomiting.
  - If your cat has vomited only a few times and <u>is otherwise behaving normally</u>, try removing access to water for 6-8 hours to see if the vomiting subsides. If vomiting continues, it is likely time to seek veterinary care.

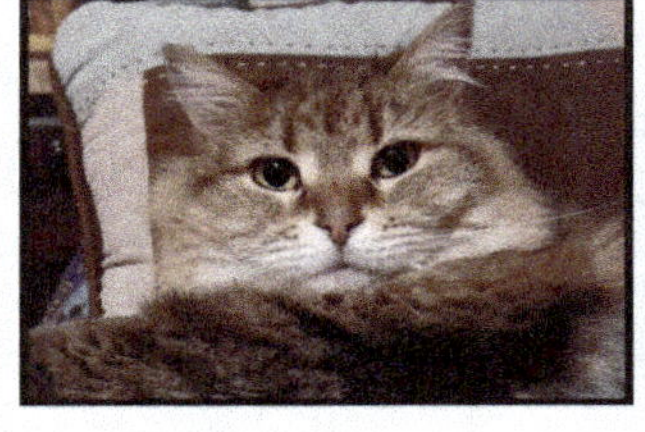

A Note About Hairballs

- Hairballs are common in cats and occur when ingested hair accumulates in the stomach and is vomited. Some cats are more prone to hairballs, particularly long-haired breeds, cats that groom excessively, or cats with underlying skin or gastrointestinal conditions.
- While an occasional hairball may be normal, it's important not to assume that vomiting is always due to hairballs. Vomiting attributed to hairballs should not be frequent, persistent, or ongoing. If vomiting occurs regularly, even if hair is present, further evaluation is recommended to rule out other causes.

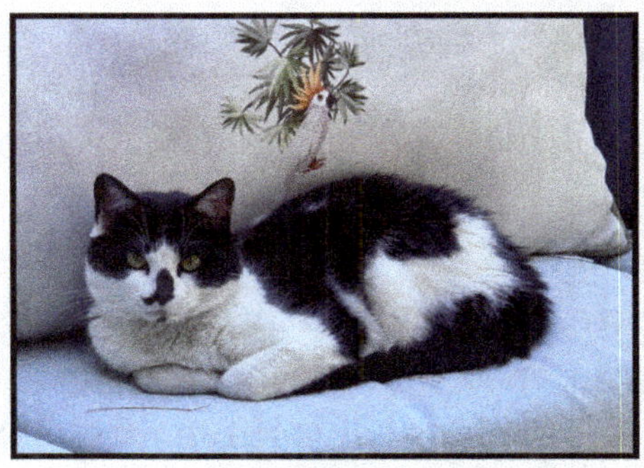

Intermittent Vomiting in Cats

Some cats may vomit intermittently, and while this is not considered normal, it can occur in certain individuals. If your veterinarian is aware of this pattern and vomiting is infrequent, they may recommend monitoring and supportive management.

However, vomiting that is accompanied by weight loss, behavior changes, decreased energy, a dull haircoat, or increasing frequency is concerning and should be investigated further. In some cases, referral to a specialist may be recommended. Advanced diagnostics such as abdominal ultrasound or sampling of the gastrointestinal tract (such as aspirates or biopsies) may be needed to evaluate for underlying disease.

<h1 style="text-align:center">Persistent Diarrhea</h1>

Loose stools that last more than a few days, especially if they are **high volume, watery, or accompanied by blood,** may indicate the need for immediate veterinary care.

Diarrhea can quickly lead to dehydration, particularly in smaller or older cats, so it's important to take these symptoms seriously.

<h2 style="text-align:center">Mild Diarrhea</h2>

Loose stools or mild diarrhea without discomfort, blood, or behavior changes are not always an emergency and may sometimes be managed at home under veterinary guidance. If your cat has recently developed loose stools but is otherwise acting normally, contact your veterinarian to discuss dietary modifications as a first step.

Bland Diet Recommendations:

- Feed boiled, unseasoned **lean protein** (such as chicken breast or turkey), finely chopped.
- Small amounts of **easily digestible carbohydrates**, such as boiled white rice, may be added.
- Avoid salt, oils, seasonings, or additives.
- Feed **small, frequent meals:**
  - Approximately 1–2 tablespoons per meal, 3–4 times daily.
- This diet should be used short-term only, unless otherwise directed by your veterinarian.
- Alternatively, a **veterinary-prescribed gastrointestinal diet** may be used in place of a home-prepared diet.

Additional Feeding Tips

- **Fiber:** Adding a small amount of plain canned pumpkin may help firm stools in some cats by increasing fiber content. Not all cats benefit from added fiber.
- **Probiotics**: Veterinary-approved probiotics formulated for cats may be recommended to support gastrointestinal health.

Dehydration can negatively impact various bodily functions. It's important to monitor for evidence of dehydration, especially if there's a known cause of fluid loss, like vomiting or diarrhea.

Below are some signs veterinarians use to assess hydration, which you can learn to check at home.

How to Check for Dehydration at Home

- **Gum Color and Moisture:**
  - Lift your cat's lip and examine the gums. Healthy gums should be **pink and moist** (See Fig 4.4).
  - If the gums feel dry or tacky, this may indicate dehydration.
    - Pale gums (See Fig 4.5) or severely reddened or purple (cyanotic) gums may be an indication of shock or further disease that requires immediate veterinary assessment.

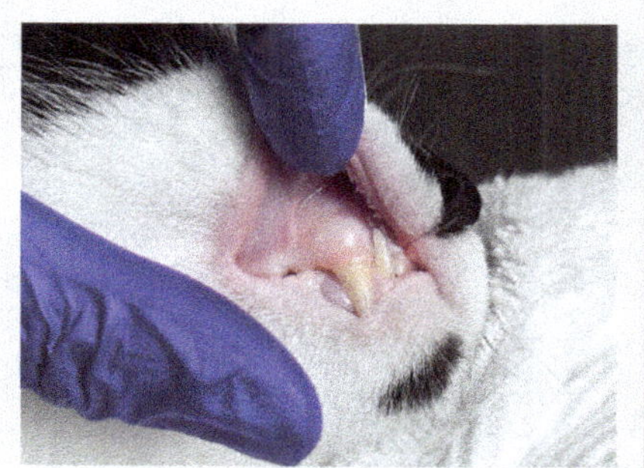

Figure 4.4: An image depicting a cat with normal pink gums

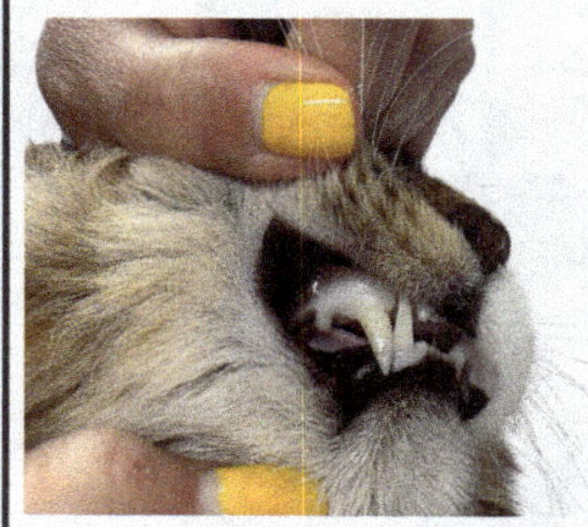

Figure 4.5: An image depicting a cat with pale and abnormal gums

- **Assessing Eye Appearance:**
  - Examine your cat's eyes. They should be bright, clear, and moist. Eyes should be comfortably seated in their sockets.
  - **Sunken** in or dull eyes may indicate dehydration.

- **Capillary Refill Time (CRT) Test:**
  - In a quiet environment, lift your cat's lip to expose the gums (See Fig 4.6).
  - Gently press on the gum area until it turns white (<1s) and then release.
    - Normal: Color returns in fewer than two seconds = good hydration.
    - Abnormal: **Prolonged (more than two seconds)** may indicate poor circulation or dehydration, which may require veterinary attention.
  - Tip: For cats with pigmented gums, check the small pink areas around the teeth or on the underside of the lip for this test (See Fig 4.7).
- *CRT test explained: The CRT test measures how quickly blood returns to the capillaries after being temporarily pushed out. In a well-hydrated cat with adequate circulation and blood volume, blood will flow quickly to the gums, and the color will return almost immediately. If your cat is dehydrated, the return of blood (and color) to the gums may be delayed.*

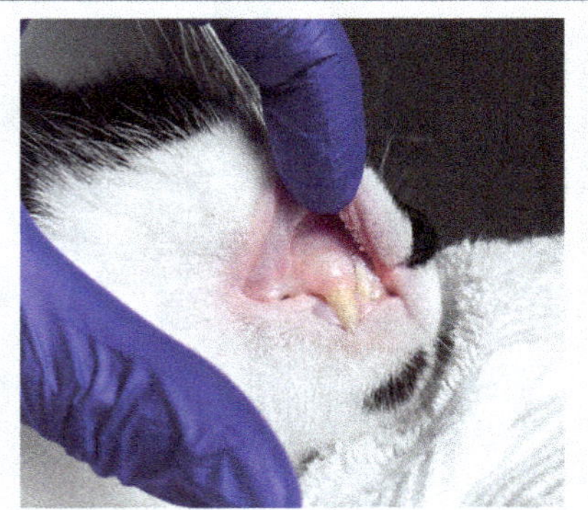

Figure 4.6. An image demonstrating positioning to check a Capillary Refill Time (CRT)

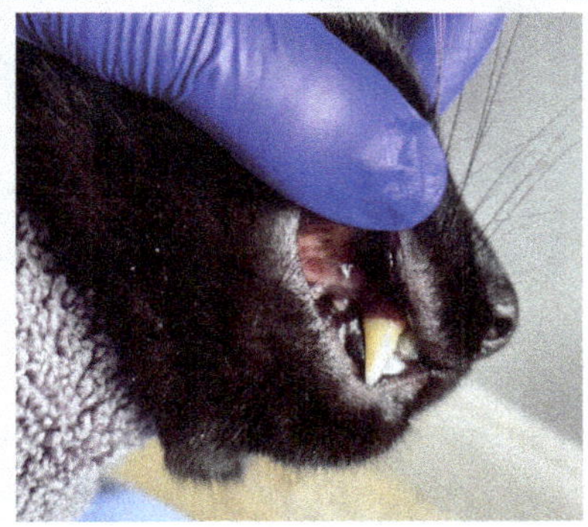

Figure 4.7. An image depicting a cat with pigmented gums. While the gums around the teeth will appear black, the underside of the lip is often pink and can be used to check gum color and CRT.

- **Skin Tenting Test:**
  - Gently pinch the skin on the back of your cat's neck or between the shoulder blades using your thumb and forefinger (See Fig 4.8).
  - Release the skin and observe how quickly it returns to normal.
    - Normal/Well-Hydrated: Skin returns to its normal position in <1 second.
    - Mild Dehydration: Skin takes 1-2 seconds to return to its normal position.
    - **Longer than two seconds:** Moderate to severe dehydration is suggested, requiring immediate veterinary care.

Skin Tenting Explained: When dehydrated, your cat's skin loses moisture and elasticity. Healthy, well-hydrated cats will have skin that is pliable and that snaps back into place immediately after being pinched. In dehydrated cats, the skin will stay tented longer due to the loss of fluid.

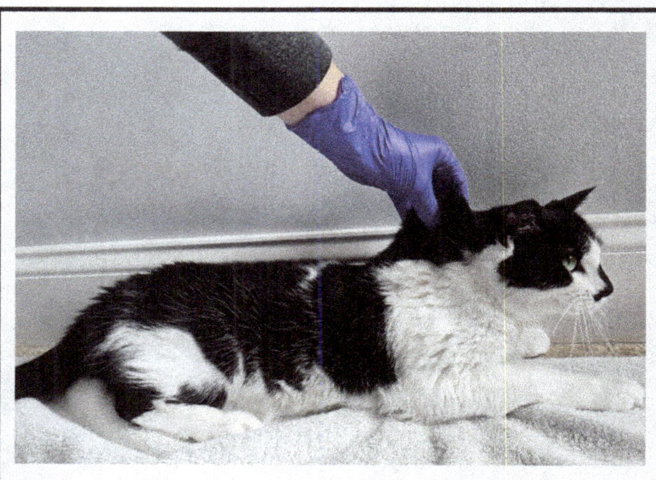

Figure 4.8. An image depicting the location and process of checking for skin tenting

Photo credit: R. Ducharme

Checking for Dehydration at Home: Practice!

Checking your cat for dehydration may seem intimidating at first, but with a little practice, it becomes a simple process. Start by getting familiar with your cat's normal condition when they're healthy. This will make it easier to spot changes later.

1. **Check Gum Color:**
   - Lift your cat's lips to examine their gums. Healthy gums should be pink (if not pigmented).
2. **Check Gum Moisture:**
   - Rub your finger on the gums. They should feel moist.
3. **Capillary Refill Test:**
   - Press gently on the gums to blanch them. Color should return in fewer than two seconds after releasing.
4. **Skin Tenting Test:**
   - Gently pinch the skin on the back of the neck or between the shoulder blades. The skin should bounce back immediately.

With practice, you'll become comfortable checking these areas and can reassess them if you have concerns.

SUMMARY:

Severe or prolonged vomiting and diarrhea in cats can be signs of serious underlying health problems that require immediate attention. By carefully monitoring your cat's symptoms and staying alert to signs of dehydration, lethargy, and other concerning behaviors, you can take swift action to protect their health. If you're ever unsure, it's always best to consult your veterinarian.

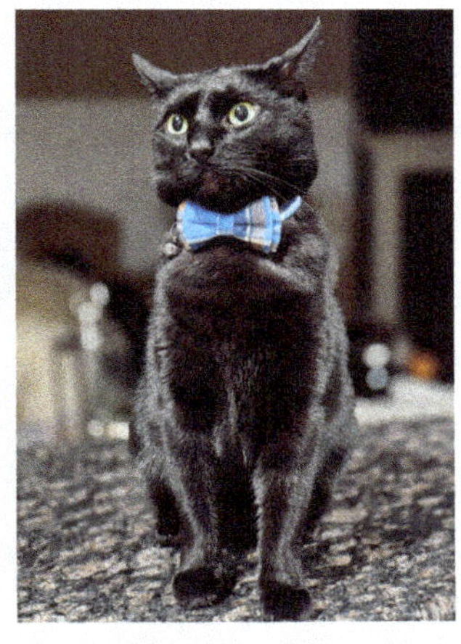

Early intervention can make a significant difference in your cat's recovery and overall well-being.

OVERVIEW

- Common Causes
- Signs
- Response
- When to Seek Care

SKILLS TOOLKIT

- Responding to a Cat in Pain
- BONUS: Pain Scales/ Scores

Possible True Emergency!

SEVERE PAIN/ DIFFICULTY MOVING

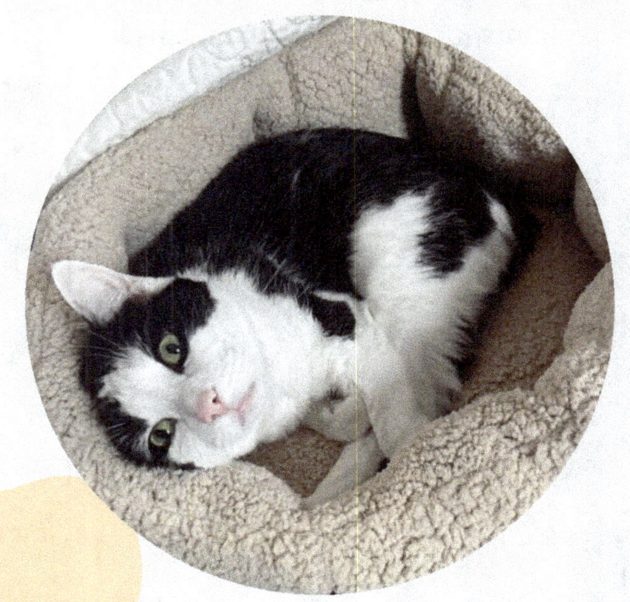

If your cat shows signs of severe pain or is having difficulty moving normally, it could indicate a serious injury or medical condition. Recognizing these signs early is critical to ensuring your cat receives the right care. Keep in mind that cats are good at hiding pain, so subtle changes in behavior and movement should not be ignored.

Common Causes of Severe Pain or Difficulty Moving

- **Injuries:** These may include fractures, sprains, or strains from accidents, falls, or rough play.
- **Joint Issues:** Conditions like arthritis or hip dysplasia can lead to chronic pain and difficulty moving.
- **Internal Conditions:** Problems such as pancreatitis, abdominal trauma, or organ rupture can cause severe pain.
- **Neurological Issues:** Spinal injuries or intervertebral disc disease can result in pain and movement difficulties.
- **Dental Pain:** Abscesses, fractures, or periodontal disease can be extremely painful but often go unnoticed.
- **Infections or Inflammation:** Infections in the abdomen, joints, or other areas can cause severe discomfort.

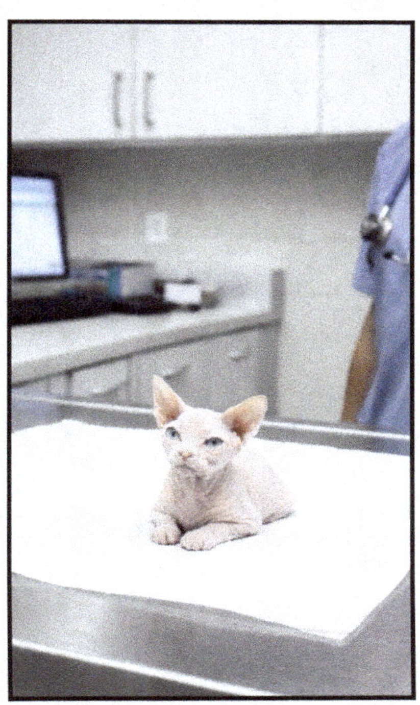

Signs of Pain

Cats express pain differently than dogs, so it's important to look for subtle signs. You may notice:

- **Vocalization:** Rare, but may include growling, hissing, or yowling (especially when touched or moved)
- **Posture**: Hunched back, holding limbs in unusual positions, or sitting/lying in a protective manner
- **Limping:** Favoring one leg or avoiding putting weight on a limb
- **Restlessness:** Pacing, hiding, or inability to find a comfortable resting position
- **Behavioral Changes:** Withdrawal, hiding, aggression when touched, or an unusual reluctance to interact with the family
- **Loss of Appetite:** Refusing food or water, which is often a sign of discomfort or illness
- **Rapid Breathing:** Increased effort or rate of breathing due to pain
- **Sensitivity to Touch:** A cat may flinch, swat, or attempt to flee if an injured area is touched.

Cats often become more withdrawn when in pain, so it's important to watch for changes in behavior, appetite, and general activity levels.

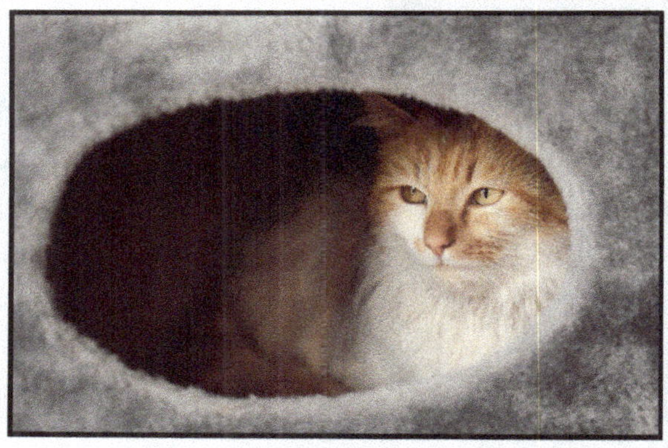

- **Limit movement.** Keep your cat in a safe, quiet, and comfortable space. Minimize handling to avoid causing more pain.
- **Assess for visible injuries.** Gently assess limbs, joints, and abdomen for swelling, heat, or tenderness. Avoid pressing on painful areas.
- **Monitor behavior.** Keep an eye on changes in eating, drinking, and overall behavior. Note whether symptoms persist or worsen over time.
- **Contact your veterinarian**. If you suspect pain or injury, call your veterinarian or an emergency clinic to describe your cat's symptoms and get advice.
- **Prepare for transport.** If transport is necessary, gently place your cat in a carrier or blanket. Keep them as still and comfortable as possible.

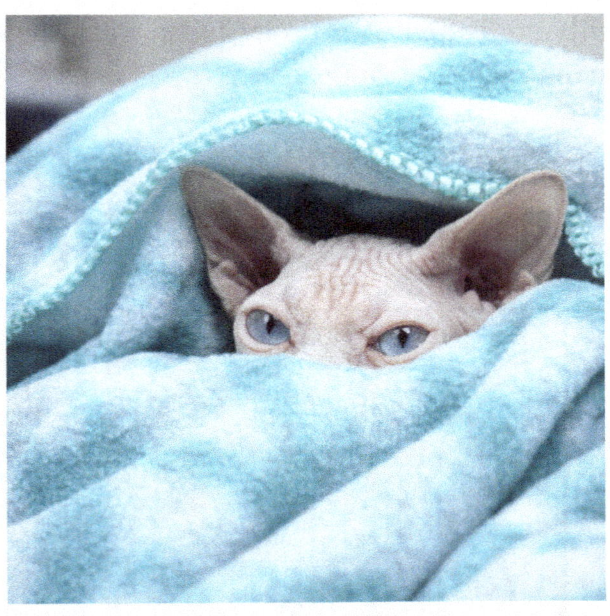

Understanding Pain Scores in Cats

A pain scale is a numerical system used to assess and quantify the level of pain an animal is experiencing. It helps veterinarians and pet owners communicate about pain levels effectively, guide treatment decisions, and evaluate treatment success.

Why Pain Scores Matter

- Cats can't verbally express their pain.
- Cats may react differently to pain, even if the severity is similar, so having a standardized scale helps owners recognize and assess it.
- Pain scales use behavioral and physical signs to categorize pain levels.

	1 Minimal Pain	**2** Mild Pain	**3** Moderate Pain	**4** Severe Pain
Behavioral signs	Subtle; Withdrawl from surroundings; Change in routine; Decreased interest in surroundings	Seeks solitude; Quiet	Unsettled; May vocalize (yowl/ growl/ hiss); Unlikely to move when left alone	Prostrate; Potentially unresponsive to surroundings; Difficult to distract from pain
Physical signs	No major changes; May exhibit mild stiffness or guarding of an area	Hunched posture; Decreased appetite; May intensively groom the painful area; Loss of brightness in the eyes	May bite or chew at an injured area; Tense muscle; Visible discomfort	Rigid; Tense posture; Reluctance to be touched (Note: Cats who do not usually seek touch may tolerate it when painful)
Cat's response to touch	May or may not react to palpation	Responds aggressively; Tries to escape; May perk up with attention	Growls/ hisses at non-painful palpation; May flinch or pull away	May not respond to palpation; May show aggression; May be rigid to avoid painful movement
Desired Intervention	Monitor. Immediate action may not be needed	Observe for worsening. Consider vet visit if pain persists	Urgent or Emergent veterinary care needed	Emergency care needed!

Figure 4.9: Feline Acute Pain Scale: Modified from CSU Guidelines

When to Seek Veterinary Care?

If your cat is experiencing significant pain or difficulty moving, seeking veterinary care is important to prevent further complications.

Seek immediate care if:
- your cat is unable to move a limb, stand, or is excessively limping.
- pain is severe or persistent.
- you notice visible injuries, swelling, or bruising.
- there is a behavioral change such as aggression when touched, hiding, or not eating.
- pain worsens over time or persists for more than a few hours.

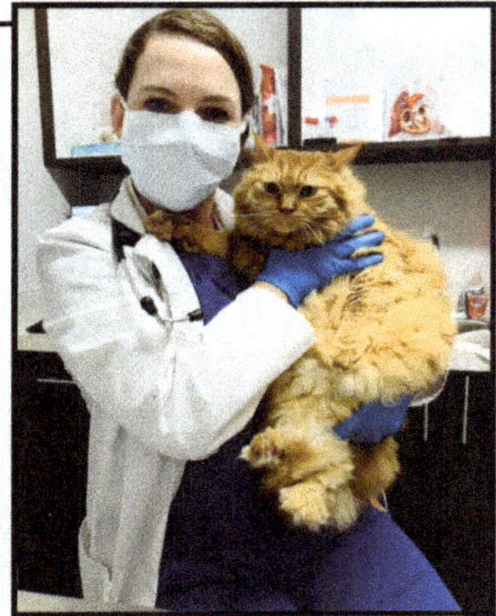
Photo credit: Dr. S. Boston

SUMMARY:

Severe pain or difficulty moving in cats can have many causes, from injuries to underlying health conditions. Cats often hide their discomfort, so subtle changes in behavior or mobility should always be taken seriously. Recognizing the signs of pain and seeking veterinary care promptly can prevent further complications and ensure that your cat gets the treatment they need. If you're unsure whether your cat is in pain, it's always better to seek professional evaluation.

OVERVIEW

- Lethargy
- Weakness
- Causes
- When to Seek Care

True Emergency!

PROFOUND LETHARGY/ WEAKNESS

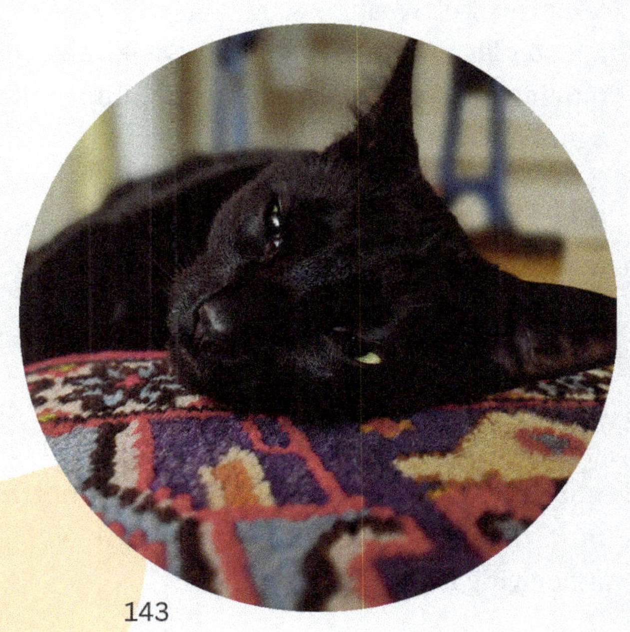

As a pet parent, it's important to be familiar with your cat's normal activity and behavior. Cats are naturally independent and curious, so any sudden change in their energy levels or activity can be a red flag. If you notice your cat becoming unusually lethargic or weak, such as refusing to stand, walking unsteadily, or even collapsing, this could signal a serious health issue that requires immediate veterinary attention.

Lethargy

Lethargy refers to a noticeable decrease in your cat's usual energy. Cats may appear unusually tired, sluggish, or weak. While some tiredness after play or activity is normal, sudden or prolonged lethargy is concerning and should be addressed promptly.

Lethargy can make a cat seem less engaged, withdrawn, or reluctant to move. They might avoid interacting or be less responsive to their surroundings.

General Weakness

Weakness refers to a lack of physical strength that may affect your cat's ability to stand, walk, or jump. It can sometimes look like lethargy, but weakness may also be caused by pain, discomfort, or neurological issues. General weakness can prevent a cat from moving properly, causing them to limp, appear unsteady, or not use a limb properly.

While lethargy primarily impacts energy and activity levels, general weakness is more related to physical strength and mobility.

Lethargy vs. General Weakness

Though lethargy and weakness are different, they can often look similar to owners, and it can be difficult to tell them apart. Both require veterinary attention. If you notice either behavior, it's important to take your cat to the vet, as both could signal underlying health issues.

Lethargy in cats can result from a variety of causes, ranging from mild to serious. These include:

- **Benign causes:** Mild viruses, tiredness from exertion, or stress
- **Pain**: Injury, discomfort, or chronic conditions like arthritis
- **Infections:** Bacterial, viral, or parasitic infections affecting various body systems
- **Toxins or Poisoning:** Exposure to harmful substances (plants, chemicals, medications)
- **Systemic illnesses**: Conditions that affect the body as a whole (e.g., kidney or liver disease, heart problems)
- **Stress or Anxiety:** Changes in environment, routine, or emotional stress
- **Chronic conditions:** Long-term health issues like hyperthyroidism or diabetes

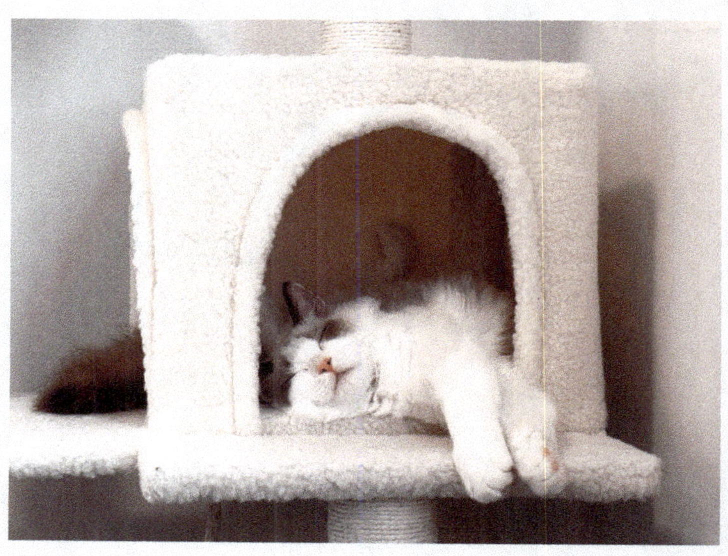

- **Lethargy lasting more than 24 hours:**
  - If your cat's lethargy persists for more than a day, it warrants a visit to the veterinarian. Prolonged lethargy is not normal, and it could point to a serious health issue.
- **Refusal to stand or walk:**
  - If your cat is suddenly unable or unwilling to stand or walk, it may signal severe weakness or discomfort. This is especially concerning if they are normally mobile or active.
- **Poor responsiveness:**
  - Cats are typically curious and energetic, but if your cat fails to respond to their name, doesn't acknowledge you, or seems disoriented, this is a sign that immediate veterinary care is needed.
- **Wobbly or unsteady gait/movement:**
  - If your cat is having difficulty walking or is unsteady on their feet, and this is combined with lethargy, it could indicate something more serious. Issues like neurological problems or severe weakness could be at play.

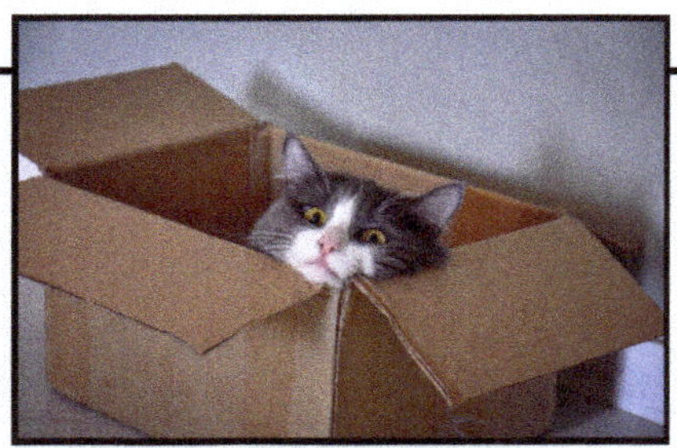

SUMMARY:

Lethargy or general weakness in cats can signal a variety of underlying health issues, from mild to serious. While it may be difficult to tell the difference between the two, both require prompt veterinary attention. If your cat is unusually tired, unresponsive, or unable to move, don't wait — seek veterinary care right away. Early intervention is crucial for your cat's recovery and well-being.

OVERVIEW

- Definitions: Tremors/ Muscle Fasciculations/ Seizures
- Order of Urgency
- When to Seek Care

SKILLS TOOLKIT

- Tremor/ Seizure Response

True Emergency!

TREMORS/ SEIZURES

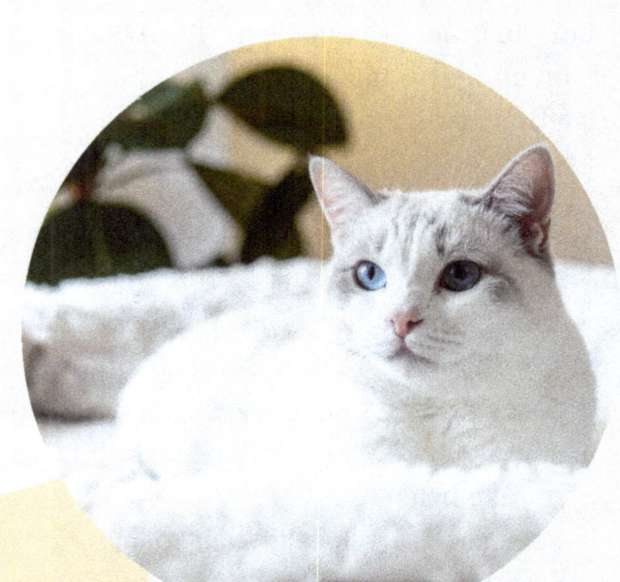

Tremors and seizures are both neurological signs that can indicate serious health concerns in cats. While they might seem similar, it's important to understand the differences and how to respond appropriately.

What are Tremors?

Tremors are **involuntary, rhythmic muscle movements** that typically affect the limbs, head, or body. Tremors can range from mild shaking to more severe and constant movements, and they can be caused by a variety of factors.

- Mild tremors may occur in response to stress, excitement, or cold temperatures.
- Severe tremors could indicate an underlying health issue, such as neurological problems or toxin exposure.

What are Muscle Fasciculations?

Muscle fasciculations are different from tremors and involve involuntary twitching or contractions of individual muscle fibers. They usually don't involve the whole body and are often localized to a particular area.

Fasciculations typically originate from the muscle itself rather than from the brain or spinal cord like tremors. They are a different type of involuntary movement and may occur due to local muscle irritation or nerve dysfunction.

What are Seizures?

A seizure is a sudden burst of abnormal electrical activity in the brain that can lead to involuntary muscle contractions, loss of consciousness, and uncontrolled body movements. Seizures usually last from a few seconds to several minutes.

- Seizures are more severe than tremors and often involve a complete loss of control, including convulsions and possible unresponsiveness.
- Seizures are typically caused by neurological issues, toxins, or systemic illnesses such as hypoglycemia or brain injury.

Common Causes of Tremors:

- Stress or excitement
- Toxin exposure: e.g., Permethrin (dog flea medication)
- Neurological issues
- Hypoglycemia
- Pain

Common Causes of Muscle Fasciculations:

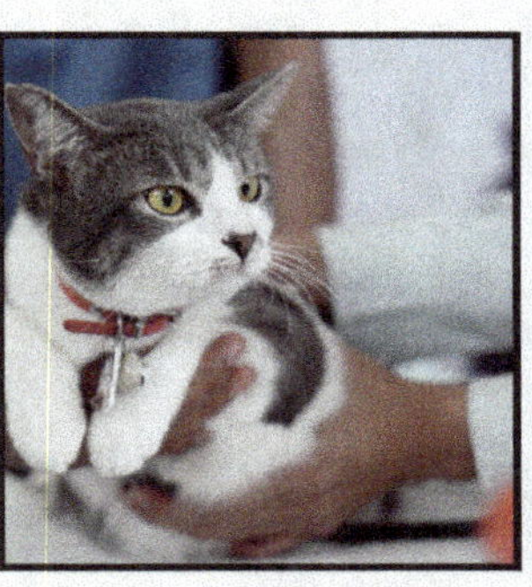

- Muscle fatigue
- Nerve irritation or injury
- Chronic diseases
- Idiopathic (no cause found)

Common Causes of Seizures:

- Infectious diseases
- Underlying brain disease (tumors, inflammation, infection)
- Toxins
- Metabolic disorder/ Systemic disease
- Head trauma
- Epilepsy (less common)

Level of Concern

- **Muscle Fasciculations**: Low to moderate concern; usually caused by muscle fatigue or nerve irritation. Should be evaluated if persistent or accompanied by other symptoms.
- **Mild Tremors:** Low concern IF temporary and linked to stress, excitement, or cold.
- **Persistent or Severe Tremors:** Higher concern; could signal neurological issues or toxin exposure.
- **Seizures:** Immediate concern; less common in cats than dogs and often associated with an underlying medical problem. Veterinary evaluation is important even after a single episode.

What to Do if Your Cat Has a Tremor or Seizure

If your cat experiences tremors:

- **Monitor** the severity and duration. If the tremors are mild and temporary (due to stress, excitement, or cold), they will usually stop once the underlying cause is resolved.
- **Keep your cat safe** in a secure space, away from sharp objects or other hazards.

If your cat has a seizure:

- **Keep your cat safe** by clearing the area to avoid injury.
- **Time the seizure.** If it lasts more than five minutes or if multiple seizures occur in a row, seek immediate veterinary care.
- **Do not try to restrain your cat** or put anything in their mouth.

When to Seek Veterinary Care

Seek veterinary care immediately if you observe:
- **Seizures:**
  - First time seizure, even if brief
  - Seizure lasting more than five minutes
  - Multiple seizures in a 24-hour period
- **Persistent or Severe Tremors:**
  - Persistent tremors
  - Tremors accompanied by neurological symptoms, such as uncoordinated movement or difficulty walking
- **Muscle Fasciculations:**
  - Usually do not require emergency care
  - If fasciculations are persistent or severe, especially when accompanied by other neurological symptoms (e.g., uncoordinated movement, disorientation), they should still be evaluated by your vet.

SUMMARY:

Tremors, muscle fasciculations, and seizures are involuntary muscle movements that can indicate underlying health issues in cats. Tremors are rhythmic shakes, often caused by stress or cold, but persistent or severe tremors may point to neurological problems or toxins. Muscle fasciculations are localized muscle twitches, typically due to muscle fatigue or nerve irritation, but they can also signal other concerns if persistent. Seizures, which involve abnormal brain activity leading to uncontrolled movements and altered awareness, are more serious and require immediate veterinary care.

Even a single seizure that stops on its own should be discussed with a veterinarian, as seizures in cats are often linked to underlying medical conditions rather than primary epilepsy. Immediate emergency care is needed if a seizure lasts more than 5 minutes, happens repeatedly, or your cat does not return to normal behavior afterward.

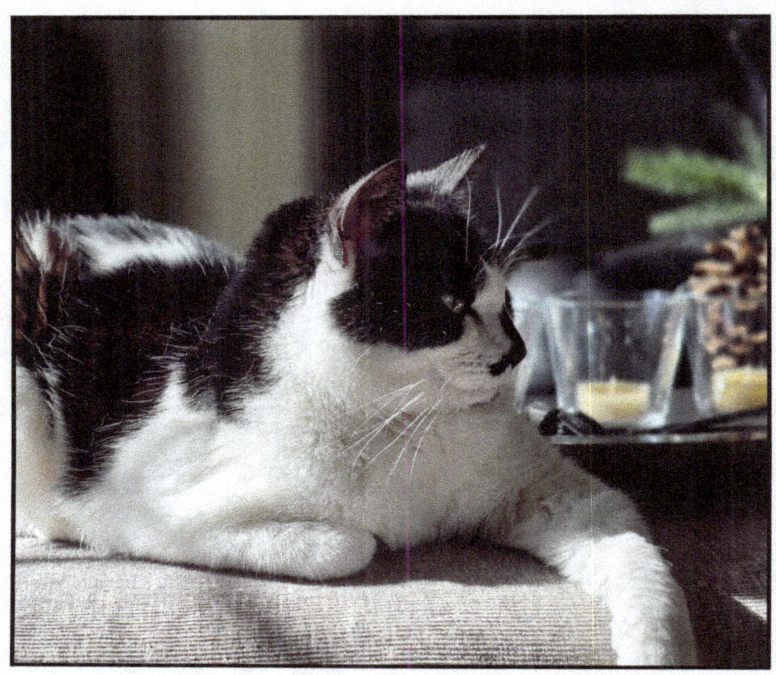

OVERVIEW

- Causes
- Signs
- When to Seek Care

Urgency/ Possible Emergency

ACUTE BLINDNESS

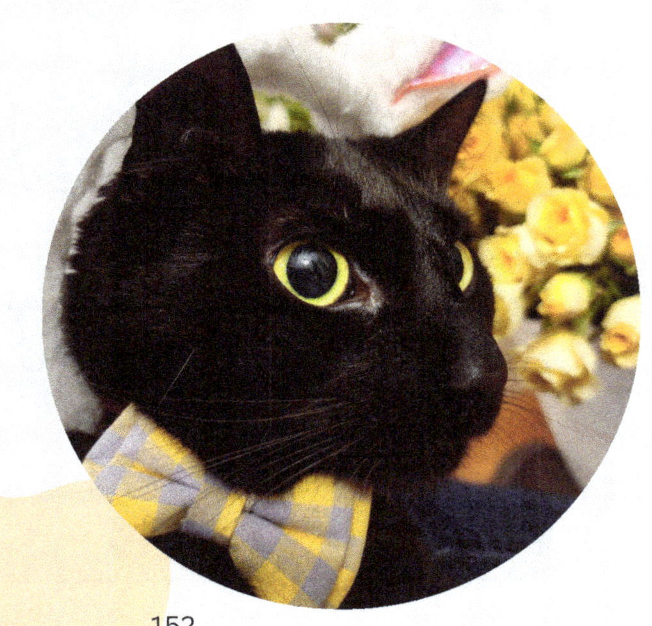

Acute blindness refers to a sudden, often dramatic loss of vision. This condition can occur very quickly, and its onset may be so rapid that the cat might appear disoriented, bumping into objects or appearing generally confused.

Common Causes:

- **Hypertension (High Blood Pressure):**
    - The rapid onset of blindness may be due to retinal detachment or bleeding in the retina.
    - This is often seen in cats with renal disease, hyperthyroidism, or heart disease. The blindness can occur in both eyes quickly.
- **Retinal Disease:**
    - Conditions such as retinal degeneration or retinal hemorrhage can cause gradual vision loss, but in severe cases, it can be acute.
    - It can affect one or both eyes, depending on the nature of the disease.
- **Glaucoma:**
    - This typically affects one eye and results in blindness due to increased pressure within the eye.
    - The onset can be rapid and severe, leading to loss of vision in the affected eye.
- **Diabetes:**
    - In diabetic cats, diabetic retinopathy can cause progressive vision loss, often starting in both eyes.
    - This usually happens more gradually.
- **Trauma:**
    - Injury to the eye, such as scratches or blunt force, can cause sudden blindness in one or both eyes, depending on the extent of the injury.
- **Toxins:**
    - Certain toxins or medications can cause sudden blindness, typically in both eyes.

Signs of Acute Blindness

When a cat experiences sudden vision loss, they may display several signs that indicate a problem with their eyesight. Common signs include:

- Disorientation
- Squinting or dilated pupils
- Reluctance to move
- Excessive sleeping or changes in behavior

What to Do if You Suspect Acute Blindness

Acute blindness warrants a veterinary evaluation.

- **Monitor** your cat's behavior closely for signs of disorientation, such as bumping into objects or difficulty moving.
- **Keep your cat safe** by removing any hazards in the environment, such as stairs or sharp objects, to prevent accidents.
- **Limit movement**: If your cat seems disoriented or hesitant, allow them to rest in a safe, familiar space.
- **Contact your veterinarian** as soon as possible.
  - They will perform an eye exam and may check for underlying conditions like hypertension, retinal disease, or toxins.
  - If your veterinarian is not available, an urgent care or emergency visit is warranted.

When to Seek Veterinary Care

You should seek immediate veterinary care if:
- you **suspect sudden blindness**, accompanied by disorientation, reluctance to move, or difficulty navigating.
- you notice your cat's **pupils are bilaterally dilated** or seem to be in **pain**.
- you suspect **toxin exposure** (e.g., flea medication, antifreeze, etc.) as a potential cause of blindness.
  - Contact poison control immediately for advice on managing exposure.
  - ASPCA Poison Control: 1-888-426-4435
- there are noticeable **behavioral changes**, such as increased lethargy or withdrawal from usual activities.

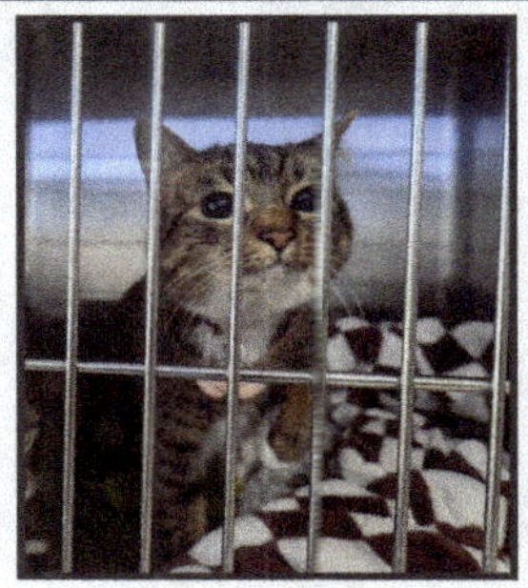

SUMMARY:

Tremors, muscle fasciculations, and seizures are involuntary muscle movements that can indicate underlying health issues in cats. Tremors are rhythmic shakes, often caused by stress or cold, but persistent or severe tremors may point to neurological problems or toxins. Muscle fasciculations are localized muscle twitches, typically due to muscle fatigue or nerve irritation, but they can also signal other concerns if persistent. Seizures, which involve loss of consciousness and uncontrolled movements, are more serious and require immediate veterinary care if they last more than five minutes or occur multiple times in a 24-hour period. If any of these symptoms occur, seeking veterinary evaluation is important to address potential health concerns.

PREVENTING EMERGENCIES

While emergencies can never be completely eliminated, many can be prevented with thoughtful planning, routine care, and close observation. Cats are masters at hiding illness and discomfort, which means problems can progress quietly before an emergency occurs. By focusing on preventive care, maintaining a safe environment, supporting a healthy weight, and monitoring daily habits, you can significantly reduce your cat's risk of serious health crises.

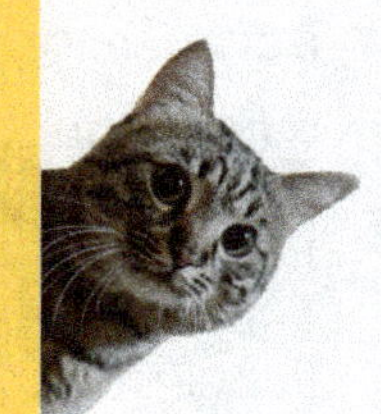

Chapter Highlights

1. Why Prevention Matters
2. Routine Veterinary Care
3. Vaccinations & Parasite Prevention
4. Healthy Weight, Nutrition, and Hydration
5. Creating a Safe, Cat-Proof Home
6. Outdoor Safety

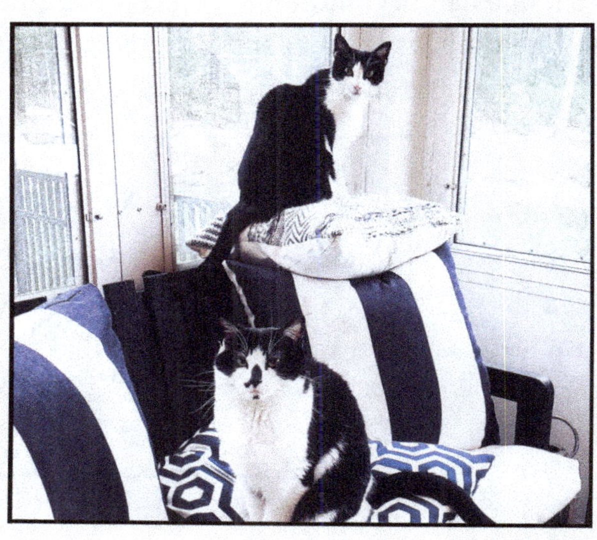

Cats are remarkably skilled at hiding illness and discomfort. In the wild, showing weakness can make an animal vulnerable, and that instinct remains strong in our companion cats today. As a result, many cats may continue eating, interacting, and behaving normally even while a medical problem is developing beneath the surface.

Because of this, emergencies in cats often appear suddenly, even when the underlying condition has been present for some time without obvious outward signs.

Preventive care plays a critical role in reducing the risk of these emergencies. Prevention is not about eliminating every possible risk, but about staying proactive, observant, and prepared. Small, consistent efforts can make a meaningful difference in a cat's long-term health and reduce the likelihood of a sudden medical crisis.

Conditions That May Develop With Minimal Outward Signs

Some common feline health conditions can progress quietly, with subtle or no visible changes at home until the disease is advanced. Some commonly encountered examples include:

- Kidney Disease
- Diabetes Mellitus
- Heart Disease
- Dental Disease
- Urinary Tract Disease

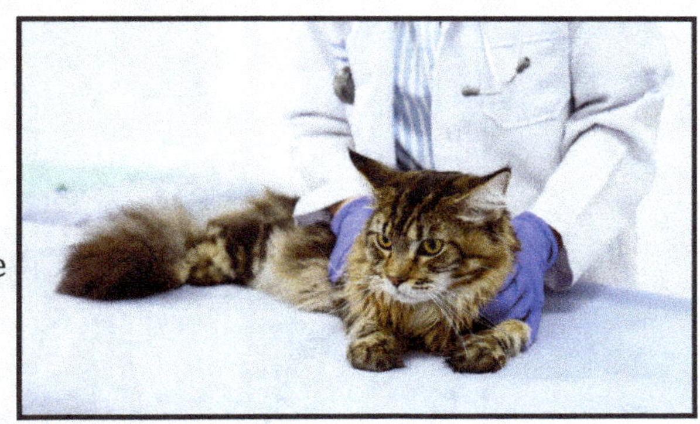

Core Components of Preventive Care

Preventive care focuses on reducing risk and identifying concerns early, before they escalate into emergency situations. Some areas where owners can have a meaningful impact include:

- Routine veterinary checkups
- Maintaining a healthy weight
- Proper nutrition and hydration
- A safe, cat-friendly home environment
- Ongoing monitoring of daily habits

These key areas provide a strong foundation for your cat's long-term health and will be explored further in the following sections.

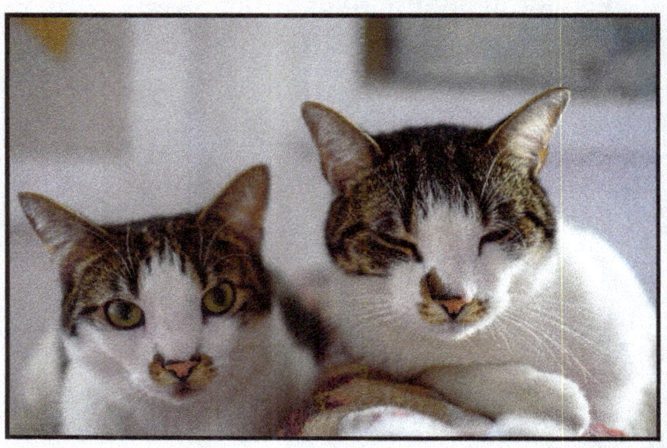

Preventive care is especially important in cats because of their remarkable ability to hide illness and discomfort. While emergencies cannot be fully prevented, attention to routine care, daily habits, and environmental safety can make a significant impact. By focusing on areas where risk can be reduced and problems can be identified earlier, owners can help support long-term health and decrease the likelihood of sudden medical emergencies.

Routine veterinary care is an essential part of preventive health, even when a cat appears healthy. Cats often hide illness, and medical conditions may be developing long before obvious signs are noticed. Regular examinations allow subtle changes to be detected early and help monitor overall health over time. This is true for all cats, including those that live strictly indoors.

Veterinary Checkups

Regular veterinary exams help identify subtle changes that may not be noticeable at home. These include:

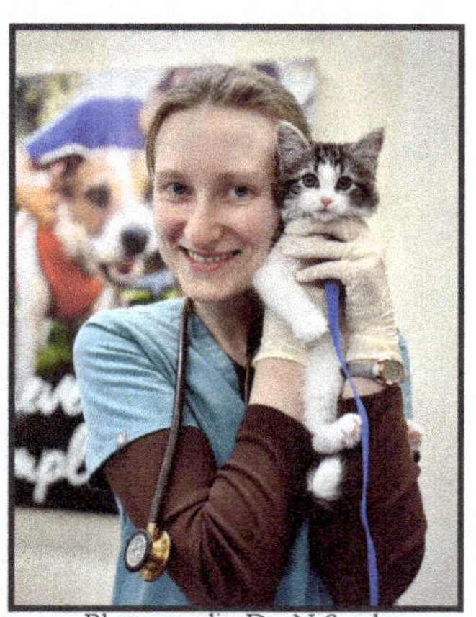
Photo credit: Dr. N Sytch

- early changes in weight, hydration, heart and lung sounds, oral health, and mobility.
- establishing baseline findings that allow changes to be recognized over time.
- identifying concerns earlier, when intervention may provide more treatment options and better outcomes.

Visit Frequency

Recommended visit schedules may vary based on age, health status, and individual risk factors.

- Younger adult cats are often examined annually.
- Older cats may benefit from more frequent visits as they age.
- Many veterinarians recommend twice-yearly exams for senior cats, often beginning around 7 years of age, though recommendations may vary.

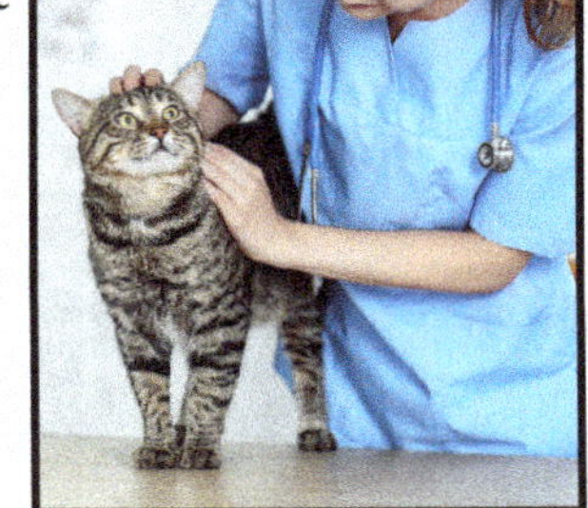

Diagnostic Screening

Routine screening tests are often recommended as they may help detect disease before obvious signs develop.

- Bloodwork can identify changes related to kidney disease, diabetes, thyroid disease, and other conditions.
- Urine testing provides valuable information about kidney and urinary health.
- Blood pressure monitoring may be recommended, particularly in older cats.
- Imaging, such as X-rays or ultrasound, may be recommended for monitoring, follow-up, or evaluating concerns about developing health changes.
- Additional testing may be advised based on exam findings.

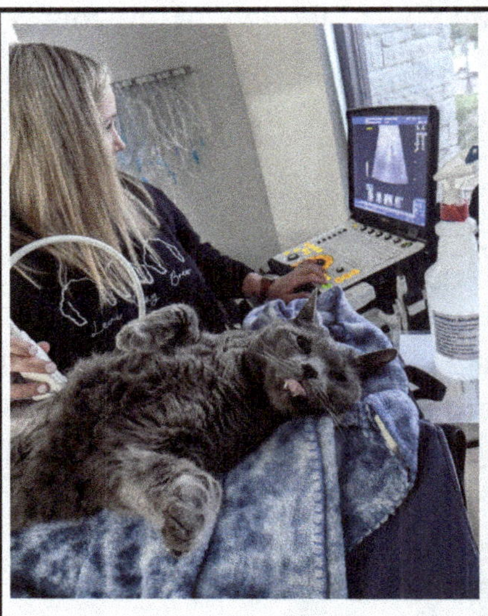

Figure 5.1. Diagnostic imaging, such as abdominal ultrasound, may be recommended to monitor, track, or diagnose health concerns.

Photo credit: Dr. B. Linchangco, with "Charlotte"

Routine veterinary care plays a critical role in identifying health concerns earlier and reducing the risk of emergencies. Even for indoor cats that appear well, regular exams and recommended screening help support long-term health and allow problems to be addressed before they become more serious.

Vaccination is an essential part of preventive care, helping protect cats from serious infectious diseases. Protection is important even for indoor-only cats, as some viruses can be carried into the home on clothing, shoes, or through brief exposures. Vaccination reduces the risk of severe illness and supports long-term health.

Vaccinations

A common misconception is that indoor-only cats do not require vaccination. While indoor living reduces certain risks, it does not eliminate them.

- Some infectious diseases can be transmitted through indirect exposure, such as on clothing, shoes, or other pets in the household.
- Cats may escape outdoors unexpectedly, even if normally kept indoors.
- Rabies vaccination is required by law in many areas and is essential for public health.
- Vaccination helps protect cats from diseases that can be severe or life-threatening.

Vaccination recommendations may vary based on age, health status, lifestyle, and local risk factors. Your veterinarian can help determine which vaccines are appropriate and how often they should be administered.

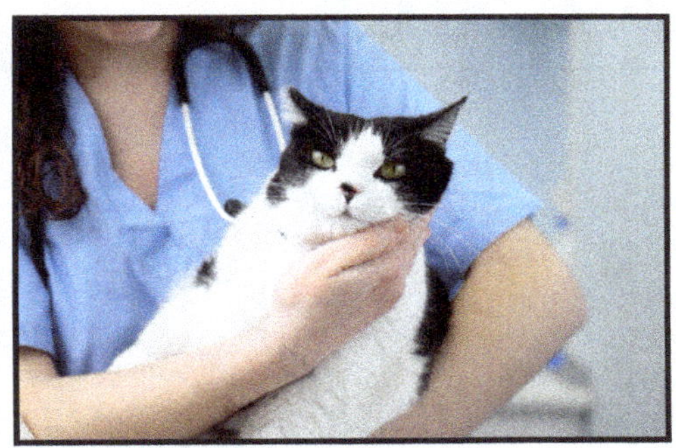

Core Vaccinations (Vaccines)

Core vaccines are recommended for most cats because they help reduce the risk of serious diseases that cats are likely to encounter over their lifetime. These vaccines include:

- **Feline Panleukopenia (FPV)**
  - Helps reduce the risk of a highly contagious viral disease that can cause severe gastrointestinal illness, immune suppression, and death.
- **Feline Herpesvirus (FHV-1)**
  - Reduces the severity and frequency of upper respiratory and eye disease related to the herpes virus.
  - Many cats are exposed at a young age and infection is lifelong once acquired. Clinical signs may not appear until later in life and can recur during periods of stress or illness.
- **Feline calicivirus (FCV)**
  - Helps decrease the risk and severity of respiratory disease and oral ulcers. Some strains may cause more severe systemic illness.
- **Rabies**
  - Rabies is a fatal disease that poses a risk to both animals and people. Vaccination significantly reduces risk.
  - This vaccine is required by law in many areas, even for indoor cats, due to public health concerns and the possibility of unexpected exposure.

Vaccination schedules and frequency may vary based on age, health status, lifestyle, and local risk factors. Vaccine recommendations and legal requirements also differ by country and region. Your veterinarian can help determine which vaccines are appropriate and how often they should be administered based on current local guidelines. If you have questions or concerns about vaccination, speaking with your veterinarian can provide individualized guidance and recommendations.

Parasite Prevention

Parasites are not limited to outdoor cats and can contribute to significant illness if left untreated.

- Fleas may be brought indoors on people, other pets, or household items.
- Flea infestations can cause skin disease, anemia, and transmission of other parasites.
- Intestinal parasites may be acquired through environmental exposure.
- Heartworm disease is transmitted by mosquitoes and, while less common in cats than dogs, can be severe and potentially fatal.

Safety Considerations:

Not all parasite prevention products are safe for cats.
- Use only products that are specifically formulated for cats.
- **Products intended for dogs (only) should never be used on cats.**
- Some over-the-counter products may not be well tolerated and, in rare cases, can result in serious adverse reactions.

Parasite prevention should be selected in consultation with a veterinarian, who can recommend products that are appropriate, safe, and effective based on individual risk factors and regional considerations.

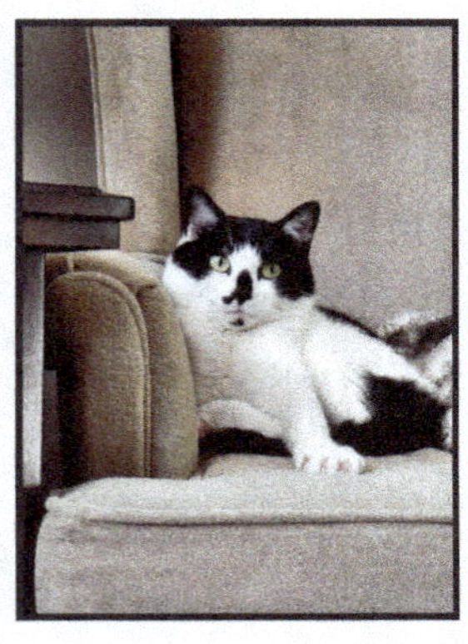

Vaccination and parasite prevention play an important role in reducing the risk of preventable disease and related emergencies in cats. Even for indoor cats, appropriate preventive care provides an added layer of protection. Working with a veterinarian helps ensure that recommendations are safe, appropriate, and tailored to each cat's individual needs.

Maintaining a healthy weight while ensuring appropriate nutrition is one of the most impactful ways to reduce the risk of emergencies and chronic disease in cats. Excess weight places strain on multiple body systems and can contribute to both short- and long-term health complications.

Health Concerns Associated with Obesity

Obesity can have a significant impact on a cat's overall health and daily comfort. While excess weight may develop gradually, it can place ongoing strain on the body and increase the risk of both chronic disease and emergency situations over time. Concerns include the following:

- Increased risk of Diabetes Mellitus
- Joint disease and decreased mobility
- Difficulty grooming, leading to skin disease and matting
- Increased risk of urinary issues
- Increased risk of constipation
- Reduced quality of life

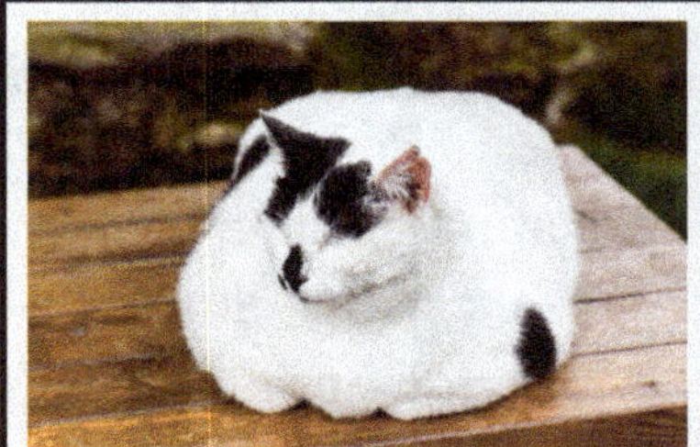

Figure 5.2. Obesity can lead to multiple health concerns in cats.

Feeding Practices and Portion Control

Feeding strategies should be tailored to the individual cat.

- Some cats are able to regulate intake when free-fed, while others are prone to overeating.
- Cats prone to weight gain often benefit from scheduled feeding.
- Portion control plays a larger role in weight management than exercise alone.

If weight gain is a concern, discuss feeding strategies and appropriate calorie intake with your veterinarian.

Encouraging Activity and Movement

While diet plays the biggest role in weight management, encouraging regular activity is also an important part of keeping your cat healthy. Not all cats are naturally active, and some indoor cats can become sedentary over time, especially as they age. Regular play and movement help keep their bodies strong, support their mental health, and reduce the risk of obesity-related issues.

Here are some ways to encourage activity:

- **Interactive play:** Engaging with your cat through toys can stimulate both their mind and body, helping them burn calories and stay active.
- **New toys:** Rotating toys regularly keeps playtime exciting and encourages physical movement.
- **Scattering food:** Placing small portions of food in different locations can inspire your cat to move around and mimic natural foraging behavior.
- **Mental enrichment:** Puzzle toys and food-dispensing toys can provide both physical and mental stimulation by encouraging your cat to "work" for their food, which satisfies natural instincts.

Incorporating these activities into your cat's routine can help them stay fit, active, and mentally engaged, promoting long-term health.

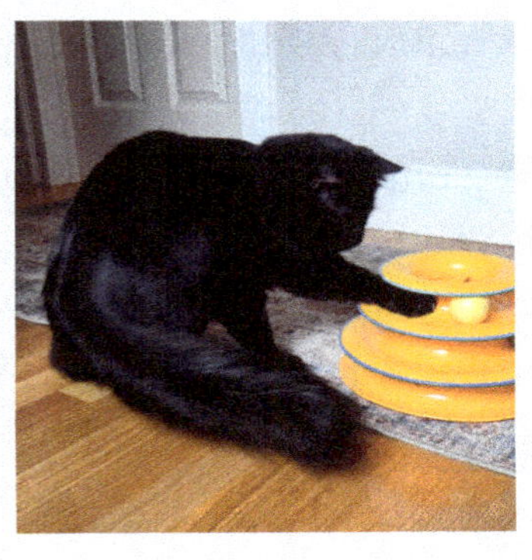

Figure 5.3. Engaging with puzzle toys can provide mental stimulation and encourage physical activity, helping to keep cats fit and active.

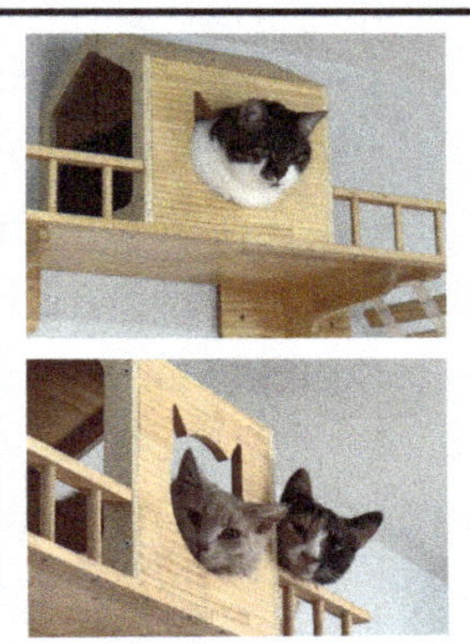

Nutrition and Hydration Considerations

Nutrition and hydration are essential to feline health and can affect both short-term well-being and long-term disease prevention.

- <u>Cats and hydration:</u> In the wild, cats get most of their hydration from their food, particularly from their prey. It's normal for cats to not drink large amounts of water, especially if they are fed wet food. As long as your cat is eating well and doesn't stop drinking altogether, this is generally not a concern.
- <u>Wet food benefits</u>: Wet food contains a high moisture content, which naturally supports hydration. Cats on wet food diets are typically better hydrated than those eating only dry food.
- <u>Introducing wet food to kittens</u>: Exposing kittens to wet food intermittently helps them become comfortable with the texture and feel of the food, making it easier for them to accept it later in life.
- <u>Hydration in senior cats:</u> As cats age, their hydration needs may increase, particularly for those with kidney disease or urinary issues. Increasing wet food intake in senior cats can support hydration and help manage these conditions.
- <u>Fresh water access:</u> It's important to ensure that cats have access to fresh, clean water at all times.
  - Some cats prefer drinking from fountains, so if you are concerned that your cat isn't drinking enough, it may be worth trying a fountain.

Dietary changes should always be discussed with your veterinarian to ensure your cat's nutritional and hydration needs are properly met, especially for those with specific health concerns.

Maintaining a healthy weight, proper nutrition, hydration, and regular activity are key to your cat's well-being. A balanced diet, fresh water, play, and a stimulating environment support their physical health, mental engagement, and long-term happiness.

A safe living space is an essential aspect of preventive care. Taking steps to remove potential hazards in the home can help prevent injuries, exposure to toxins, and other safety risks for cats. Ensuring a secure environment is key to supporting a cat's health and well-being.

Pet-Proofing Your Home

- Keep Toxic Foods and Substances Out of Reach
  - Secure harmful foods, medications, cleaning supplies, and chemicals away from reach.
- Ensure Plant Safety
  - Make sure all plants brought into the home are non-toxic to cats.
- Prevent Burns or Injuries
  - Protect your cat from hot surfaces like stoves, fireplaces, or candles. Burns from hot surfaces or open flames can be serious injuries.
- Protect from Sharp Objects/Edges
  - Items like scissors, knives, and sharp-edged furniture can cause cuts and wounds. Keep these stored safely out of your cat's reach.
- Electrical Safety
  - Cats are naturally curious and may chew on wires or cords. Cover outlets and use cord protectors to avoid electric shocks.
- Secure Trash and Food
  - Use pet-proof trash cans and avoid leaving food on counters where it's easily accessible.

Creating a safe, cat-proof home helps prevent injuries, exposure to toxins, and other safety risks. By taking these precautions, you can provide a secure environment for your cat.

If you choose to allow your cat outdoors, it's important to take certain precautions to ensure their safety. Indoor-only cats are generally safer, but outdoor access can be managed with the right precautions.

Common Outdoor Hazards

Outdoor cats face a variety of risks that should be carefully considered before granting outdoor access. These include:

- Traffic: Busy roads pose a serious risk of accidents.
- Predators: Other animals, such as dogs, wildlife, and even other cats, can be a threat.
- Diseases and Parasites: Outdoor cats are at a higher risk of diseases like FIV, FeLV, and parasitic infections like fleas and ticks.
- Toxins: Exposure to harmful substances such as antifreeze, certain plants, and chemicals can lead to poisoning.

Safer Outdoor Alternatives

While the risks are significant, there are ways to allow your cat to enjoy the outdoors safely:

- <u>Leash and Harness Training:</u> A leash and harness allow you to supervise your cat while they enjoy the outdoors, minimizing risks and providing controlled exposure.
- <u>Catios</u> (Enclosed Outdoor Spaces): Catios or secure outdoor enclosures provide a safe, enclosed area where your cat can experience the outdoors without the risks of roaming free.
- <u>Supervised Outdoor Time:</u> If you prefer your cat to have some outdoor time, always accompany them to ensure their safety and prevent them from wandering into dangerous areas.

Outdoor Cat Safety

To further ensure your cat's health and safety while outdoors, follow these precautions:

- Ensure cats are inside at night.
    - Nighttime increases exposure to predators, reduced visibility, and higher traffic. Keeping your cat indoors during the night helps reduce these risks.
- Keep vaccinations up to date.
    - Ensure your cat is up to date on vaccinations, especially for rabies. Rabies is a serious disease, and outdoor cats are at higher risk of exposure.
    - Keeping your cat's rabies vaccination current is essential for their protection and also important in case your cat bites or scratches another animal or a human.
- Check for injuries after outdoor time.
    - Always inspect your cat for bites, scratches, or signs of parasites (fleas or ticks) after they've been outside.
- Create a barrier from roads.
    - Make sure outdoor spaces are securely enclosed and located away from busy roads.
- Ensure pets are spayed or neutered.
    - Intact animals are more likely to fight, be attacked, or contribute to overpopulation.

By following these precautions, you can minimize the risks associated with outdoor access and help ensure your cat's safety in both indoor and outdoor environments.

Outdoor access for cats comes with inherent risks, but by taking certain precautions and providing safe outdoor alternatives, you can help minimize these risks.

Summary

Emergencies with our cats are bound to happen at times. We cannot fully prevent them. However, with the right knowledge and a combination of preventative measures and preparation, we can be better equipped to respond in a timely manner when these emergencies do occur. Regular veterinary care, up-to-date vaccinations, parasite prevention, proper nutrition, and a safe, cat-proof home all play important roles in supporting your cat's health and safety. By focusing on prevention, we give our cats the best chance for a long, healthy life, and we are better prepared to handle any challenges that arise.

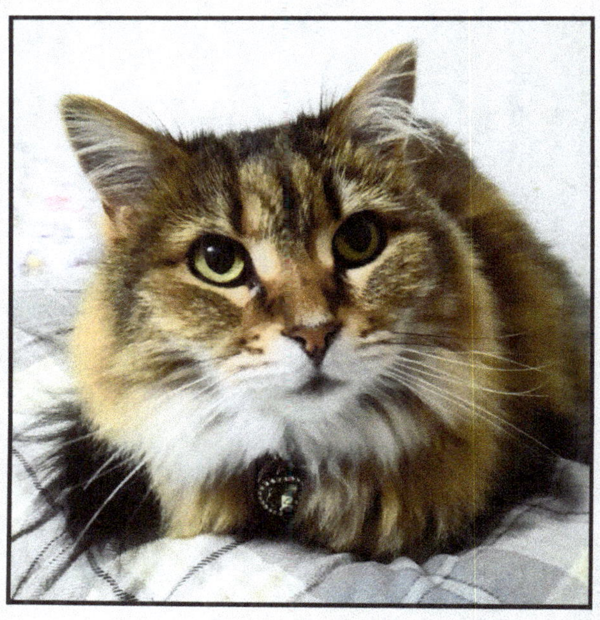

EMERGENCY TOOLKIT & RESPONSE FLOWCHARTS

What is Your Emergency Toolkit?

Throughout this book, several simple hands-on assessment tools were introduced to help you better understand your cat's condition during a health concern.

This page provides a quick reference for each tool and what they help evaluate. Use the page numbers listed below to revisit the full sections for detailed guidance.

TOOL	USED TO EVALUATE	SECTION	PAGE #
Resting Respiratory Rate	Breathing Status	Difficulty Breathing	110
Urinary Bladder Assessment	Urinary Obstruction Potential	Urinary Issues	114
Eye Assessment for Hydration	Hydration	Vomiting/Diarrhea	133
Gum Moisture Assessment	Hydration	Vomiting/Diarrhea	133
Capillary Refill Time	Hydration	Vomiting/Diarrhea	134
Skin Tenting	Circulation & Hydration	Vomiting/Diarrhea	135
Pain Scale	Comfort & Mobility	Pain/ Difficulty Moving	141

Figure 6.1: Calculating Resting Respiratory Rate

Resting Respiratory Rate (RRR):
Used to monitor your cat's breathing rate over time

Process
- Watch the chest rise and fall.
- Count the number of breaths in six seconds.
- Multiply by ten.
  - This is your cat's **breaths/minute**

Normal: Fewer than 40 breaths per minute

Figure 6.2: Palpating the Urinary Bladder

How to Palpate the Bladder at Home
Only attempt if your cat is calm and tolerates handling.

Note: The bladder may be difficult or impossible to feel in overweight cats or cats with tense abdominal muscles.

Process:
- Allow your cat to remain standing on a stable surface.
- Gently cup the lower abdomen with one hand, just in front of the hind legs.
- With your hand cupped, gently scoop backward toward the tail while lifting slightly.
  - Use very light pressure.
  - Notice what you feel.
  - Watch how your cat responds.

Normal:
- Bladder feels small and soft.
  - It may be difficult to feel when normal.
- Cat remains comfortable during gentle palpation.

Figure 6.3. Dehydration evaluation Techniques

Gum Moisture

Process
- Lift your cat's lips to examine the gums.
- Lightly run a finger across the gums to assess moisture.

Normal: Moist gums
Abnormal: Tacky gums, which may indicate dehydration

Eye Assessment

Process
- Evaluate the eyes for brightness, moisture, and position.

Normal: Bright, clear, moist eyes that sit comfortably in their sockets
Abnormal: Dull or sunken eyes

Skin Tenting

Process
- Gently pinch the skin on the back of the neck or between the shoulder blades using your thumb and forefinger.
- Release the skin and observe how quickly it returns to normal.

Normal: Skin returns to normal position in <1 second
Mild Dehydration: Skin remains tented for 1-2 seconds
Moderate/Severe Dehydration: Skin tenting for >2seconds

Capillary Refill Time (CRT)

Process:
- Expose your cat's gums. Gently press on the gum until it turns white (about one second). Then release.

Normal: Color returns in <2 seconds
Abnormal: Prolonged response of >2seconds

Figure 6.4: Observing Signs of Pain

Note: Cats rarely cry when in pain. Behavior changes are often the first and sometimes only sign.

Observe your cat at rest and during normal movement.

Look for changes such as:
- Hiding more than usual
- Reduced activity or reluctance to move or jump
- Sitting hunched or with a tucked posture
- Tense body or stiff movement
- Decreased grooming or unkempt coat
- Changes in appetite
- Growling, hissing, or avoiding interaction
- Dilated pupils in normal lighting
- Increased breathing rate while resting

Normal:
- Cat moves, rests, and interacts as usual

Concerning:
- New behavior changes, reluctance to move, or signs listed above

The next section walks through common emergency situations and possible responses, with some of the tools from this chapter included where helpful.

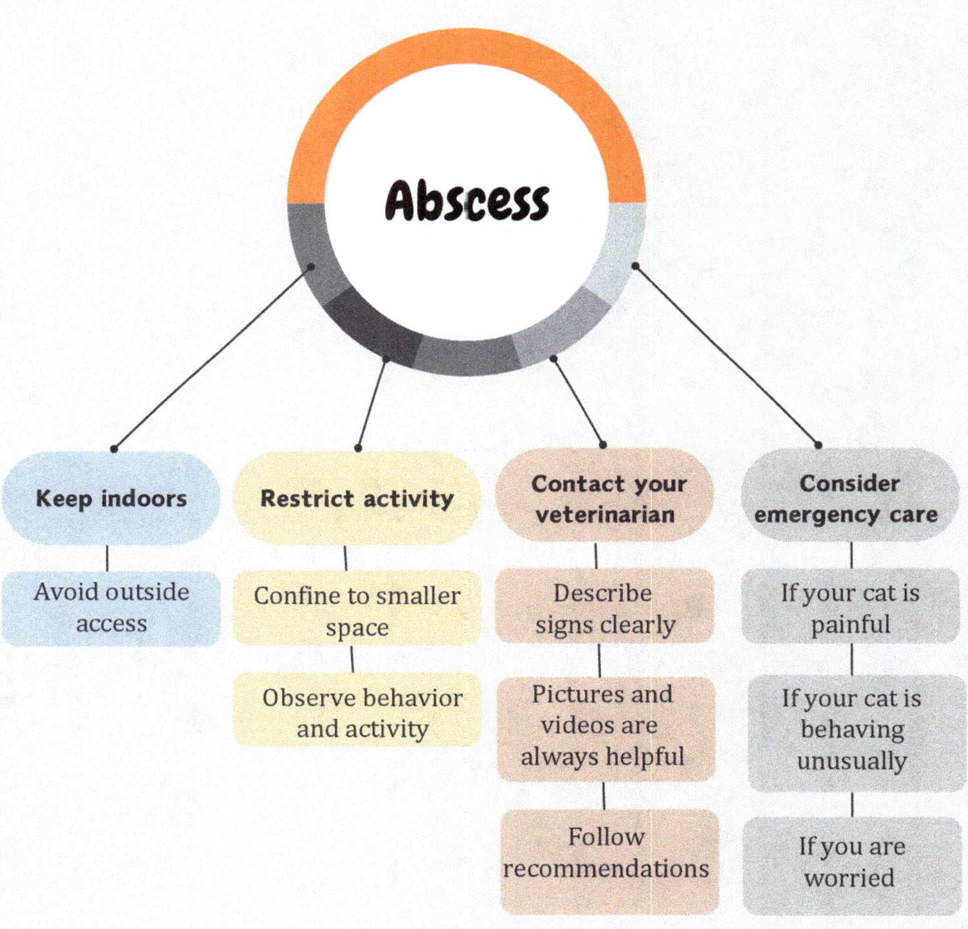

For more information, see page 15. This guide does not replace veterinary care. Seek professional care if concerns arise.

Figure 6.6. Responding to Suspected String or Ribbon Ingestion

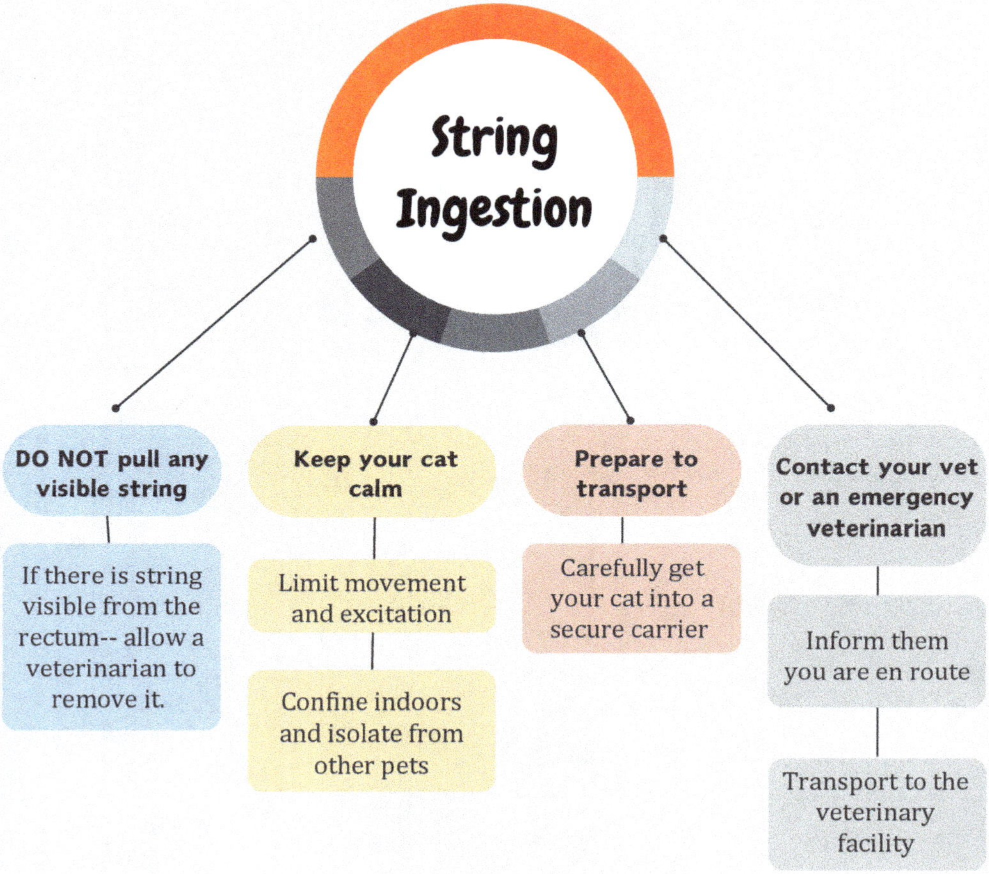
String Ingestion
DO NOT pull any visible string
If there is string visible from the rectum-- allow a veterinarian to remove it.
Keep your cat calm
Limit movement and excitation
Confine indoors and isolate from other pets
Prepare to transport
Carefully get your cat into a secure carrier
Contact your vet or an emergency veterinarian
Inform them you are en route
Transport to the veterinary facility

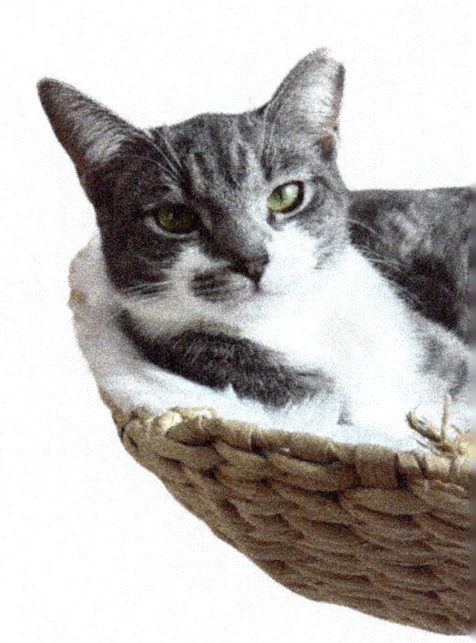

For more information, see page 19.

This guide does not replace veterinary care. Seek professional care if concerns arise.

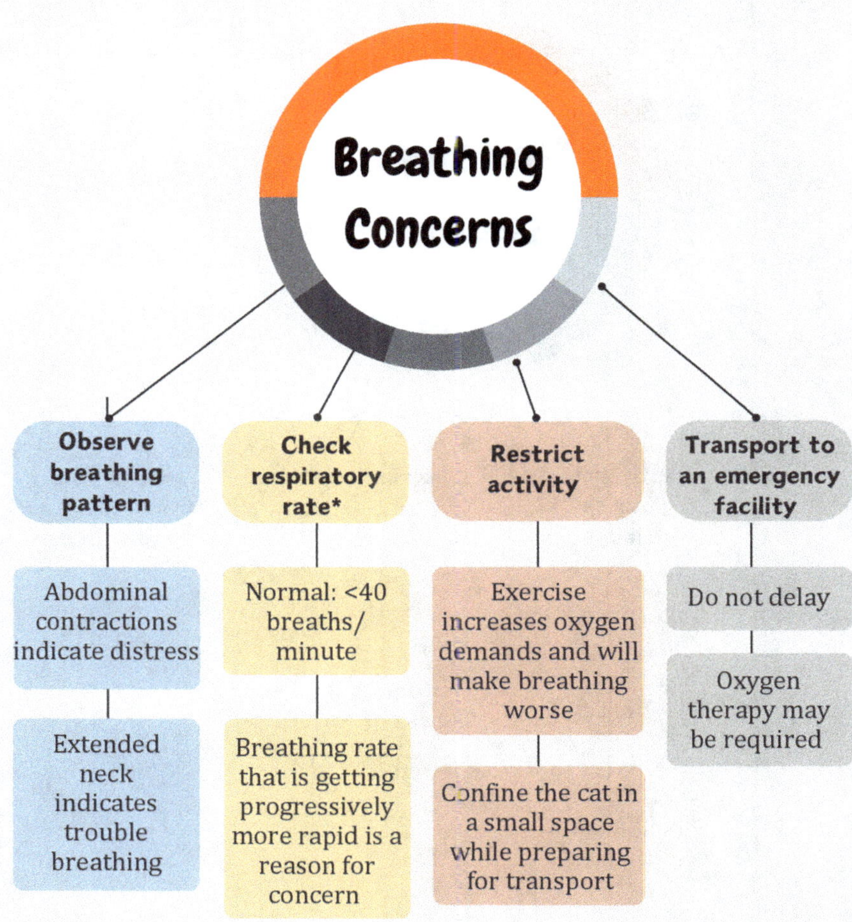

*Refer to the Difficulty Breathing section (page 109) for a tutorial on how to check respiratory rate and effort.

For more information, see pages 23 and 108.

This guide does not replace veterinary care. Seek professional care if concerns arise.

Figure 6.8. Responding to Suspected Urinary Blockage (Especially Male Cats)

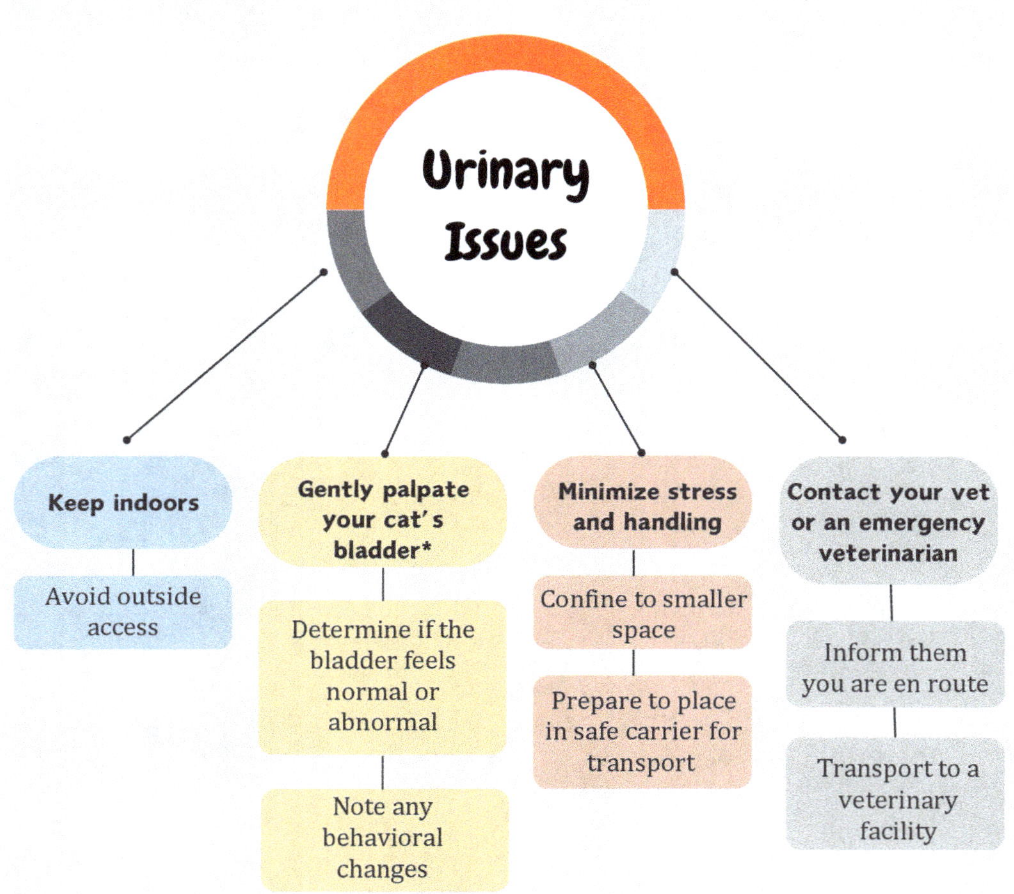

*Refer to the Bladder palpation section (page 114) for a tutorial on how to palpate urinary bladders.
NOTE: Some cats will not tolerate this.

For more information, see pages 30 and 112.

This guide does not replace veterinary care. Seek professional care if concerns arise.

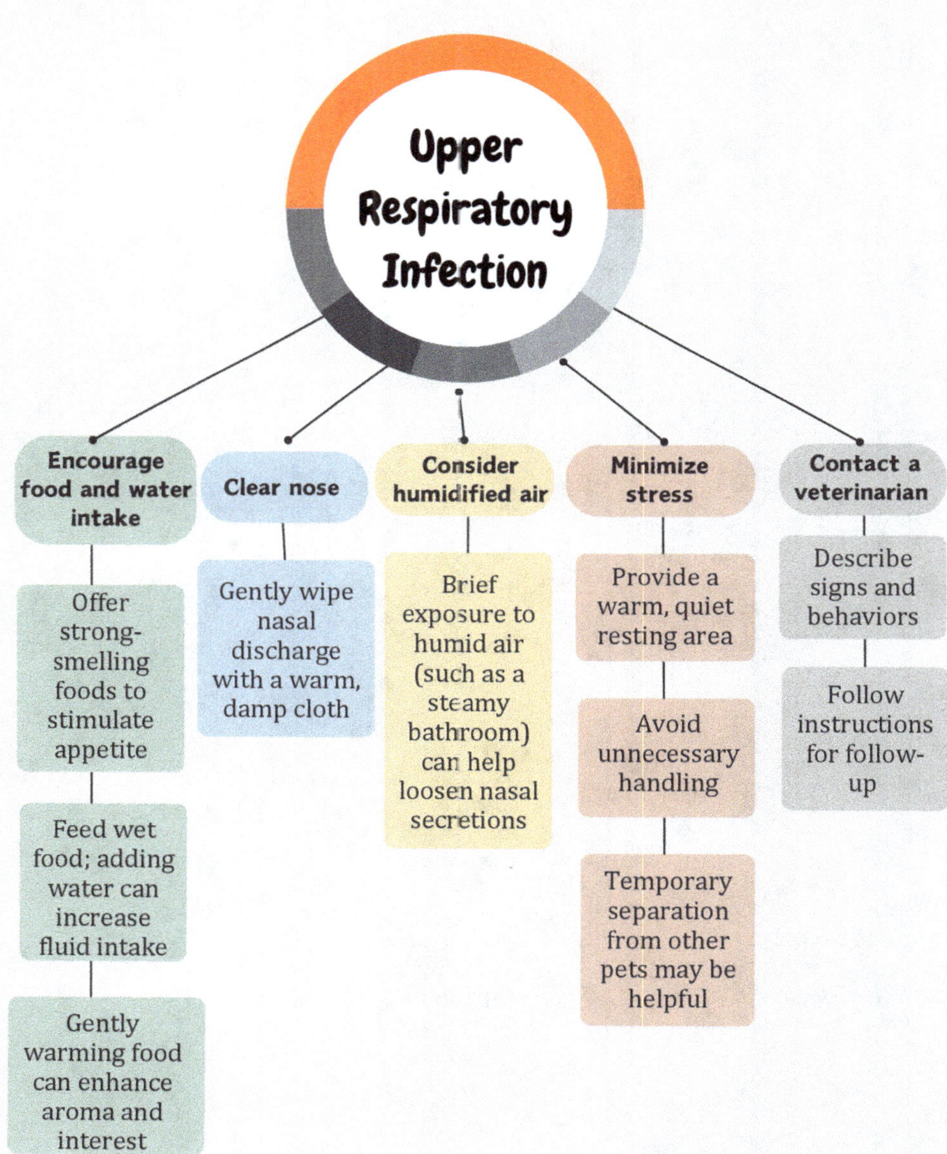

For more information, see page 54.
This guide does not replace veterinary care. Seek professional care if concerns arise.

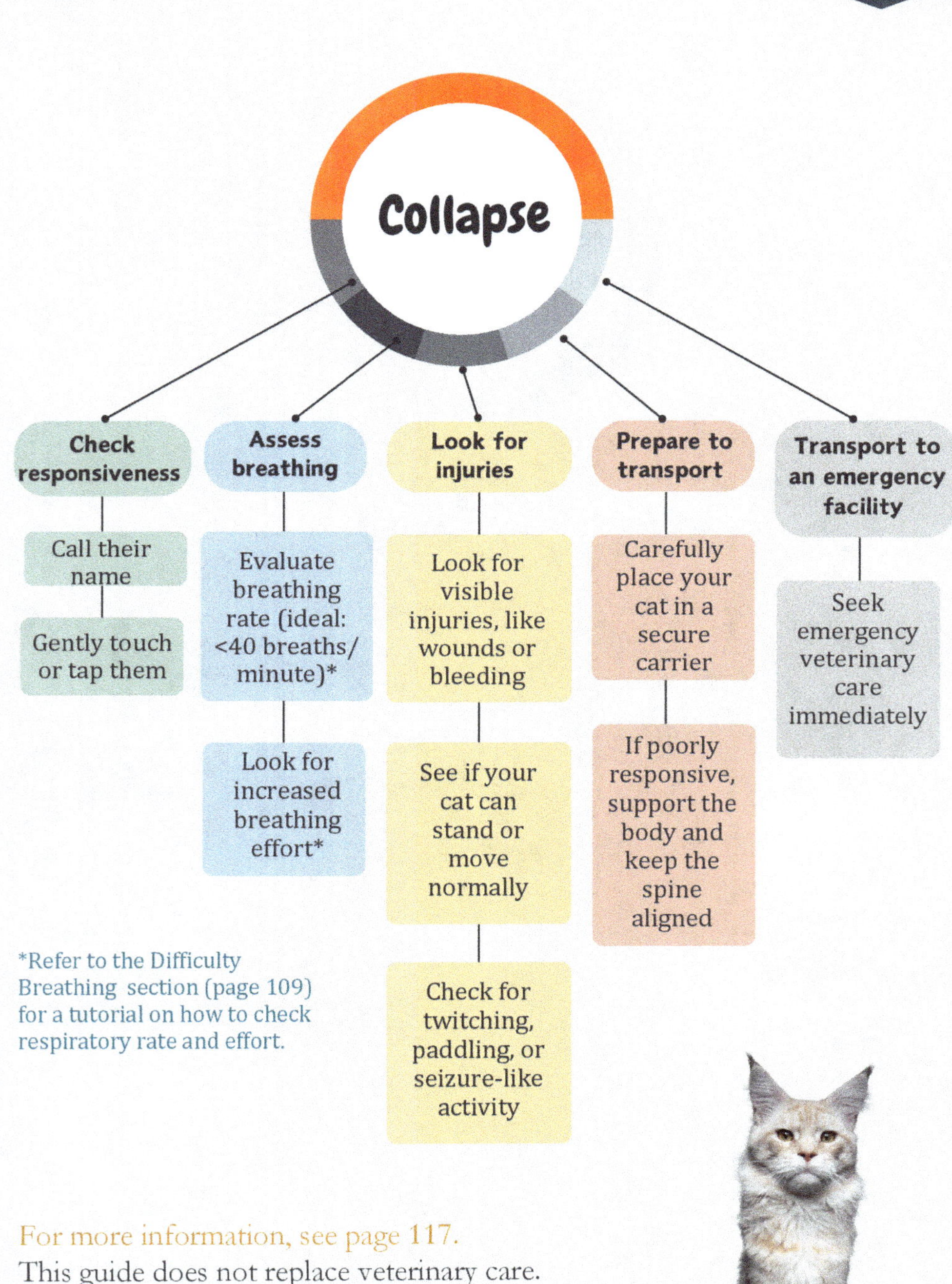

For more information, see page 117.
This guide does not replace veterinary care.
Seek professional care if concerns arise.

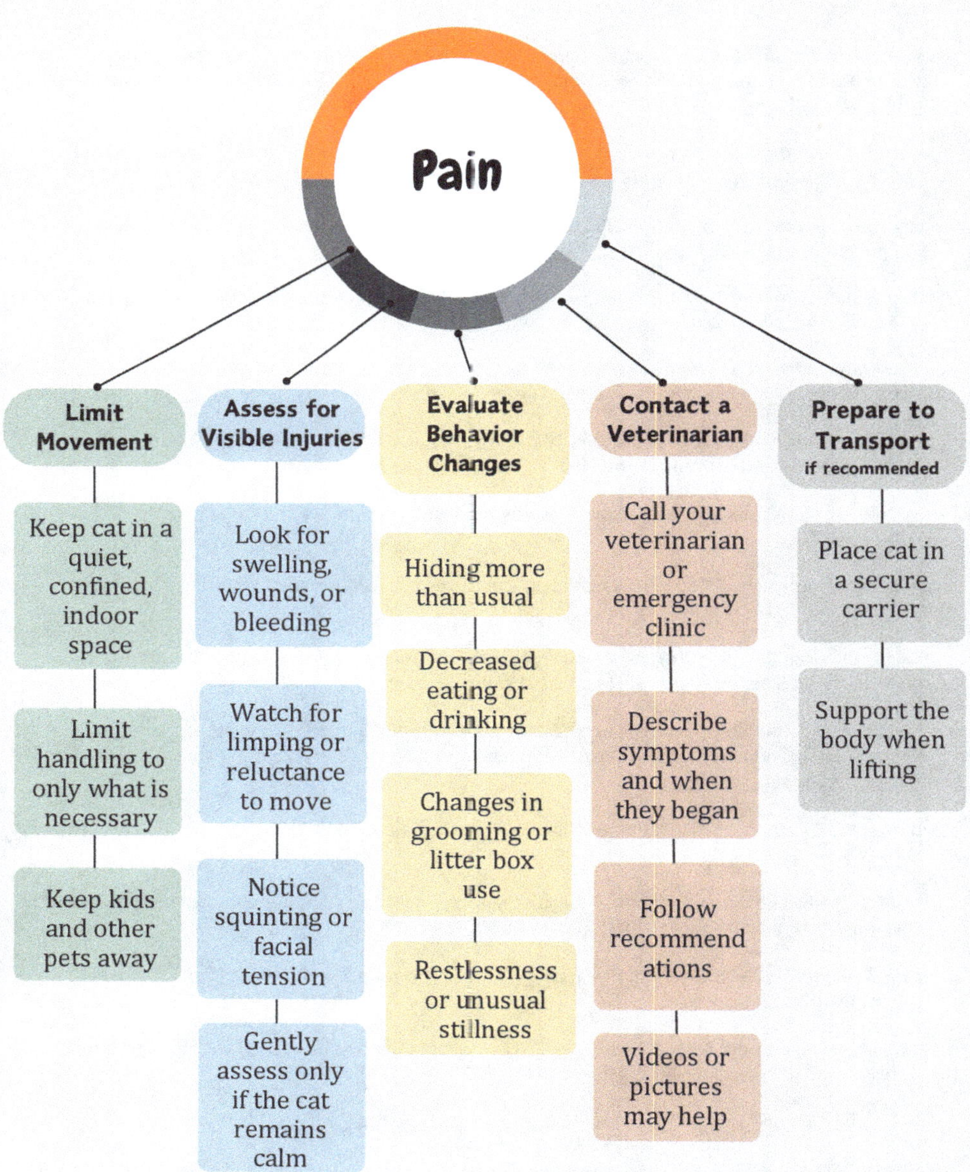

*Refer to the Pain Score chart, page 141

For more information, see page 137.
This guide does not replace veterinary care.
Seek professional care if concerns arise.

REFERENCES
& ADDITIONAL RESOURCES

American Animal Hospital Association (AAHA). (n.d.). Preventive care standards, parasite control, and vaccination principles. https://www.aaha.org

American Association of Feline Practitioners (AAFP). (n.d.). Feline preventive care guidelines, vaccination recommendations, environmental enrichment, and indoor and outdoor considerations. https://catvets.com

American Society for the Prevention of Cruelty to Animals (ASPCA) Animal Poison Control Center. (2023). Annual report of animal poisoning incidents. https://www.aspca.org

American Society for the Prevention of Cruelty to Animals (ASPCA) Animal Poison Control Center. (n.d.). Pet poisoning and toxicology. https://www.aspca.org

American Society for the Prevention of Cruelty to Animals (ASPCA) Animal Poison Control Center. (n.d.). Poison control resources for pets. https://www.aspca.org

American Society for the Prevention of Cruelty to Animals (ASPCA) Animal Poison Control Center. (n.d.). Toxic and non-toxic plants for cats and common household toxins. https://www.aspca.org

American Veterinary Medical Association (AVMA). (n.d.). Rabies vaccination, public health considerations, and preventive veterinary care. https://www.avma.org

Bates, N., et al. (2022). Suspected poisoning in dogs and cats with grapes and raisins. Veterinary Record, 190(6), e1222.

Bischoff, K., & Morgan, S. E. (2019). Essential oil exposures in cats. Journal of Veterinary Emergency and Critical Care, 29(4), 421–427.

Brown, S. A., & Henik, R. A. (2018). Systemic hypertension and target organ damage in cats. Journal of Veterinary Internal Medicine, 32(6), 1937–1950.

Cornell Feline Health Center. (n.d.). Feline health topics including nutrition, obesity, urinary disease, hypertension, and indoor safety. Cornell University College of Veterinary Medicine. https://www.vet.cornell.edu

Cortinovis, C., & Caloni, F. (2015). Epidemiology of intoxications in cats. Veterinary Record, 176(14), 372.

Court, M. H., & Greenblatt, D. J. (1997). Molecular basis for deficient acetaminophen glucuronidation in cats. American Journal of Veterinary Research, 58(4), 387–392.

Gwaltney-Brant, S. (2018). Veterinary toxicology. In M. E. Peterson & P. A. Talcott (Eds.), Small animal toxicology (3rd ed.). Elsevier.

Hall, J. O., Gwaltney-Brant, S. M., & Khan, S. A. (2014). Nephrotoxicity associated with lily ingestion in cats. Journal of Veterinary Emergency and Critical Care, 24(4), 392–398.

International Cat Care. (n.d.). Seizures in cats. https://icatcare.org

Khan, S. A., & McLean, M. K. (2012). Toxicology of commonly encountered human pharmaceuticals in pets. Veterinary Clinics of North America: Small Animal Practice, 42(2), 207–224.

Langston, C. E. (2002). Acute renal failure caused by lily ingestion in cats. Veterinary Clinics of North America: Small Animal Practice, 32(4), 925–939.

REFERENCES
& ADDITIONAL RESOURCES

Merck Veterinary Manual. (n.d.). Toxicology and poisoning topics, including chocolate toxicity, detergent toxicity, essential oil toxicity, NSAID toxicity, onion and garlic toxicity, and vitamin D toxicity. https://www.merckvetmanual.com

Papich, M. G. (2016). Saunders handbook of veterinary drugs (4th ed.). Elsevier.

Peterson, M. E., & Talcott, P. A. (2013). Small animal toxicology (3rd ed.). Elsevier.

Reassessment Campaign on Veterinary Resuscitation (RECOVER) Initiative. (2024). RECOVER evidence-based veterinary CPR guidelines. https://recoverinitiative.org

Scherk-Nixon, M., et al. (2007). Carprofen toxicosis in cats: Case report and review. Journal of Veterinary Emergency and Critical Care, 17(1), 94–99.

Vet Neuro Chesapeake. (n.d.). Feline seizures and seizure disorders in cats. https://www.vetneurochesapeake.com/diseases-cat-seizures

Veterinary Information Network (VIN). (2025). Day lily toxicosis in cats. https://www.vin.com (member resource)

Veterinary Information Network (VIN). (2025). Feline toxicology resource. https://www.vin.com (member resource)

Veterinary Information Network (VIN). (2025). Household toxins: Dogs and cats. https://www.vin.com (member resource)

Veterinary Information Network (VIN). (2025). Toxin and household exposure database. https://www.vin.com (member resource)

VCA Animal Hospitals. (n.d.). Retinal detachment in cats. https://vcahospitals.com

VCA Animal Hospitals. (n.d.). Seizures and epilepsy in cats. https://vcahospitals.com

World Small Animal Veterinary Association (WSAVA). (n.d.). Global vaccination guidelines and preventive care frameworks. https://wsava.org

Yamato, O., & Maede, Y. (1992). Susceptibility to onion-induced hemolysis in cats. Journal of Veterinary Medical Science, 54(4), 719–724.

Dr. Gal Chivvis

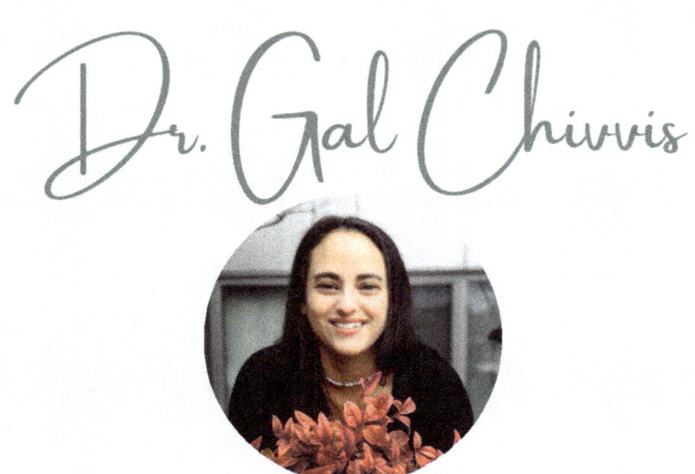

Dr. Gal Chivvis is an emergency veterinarian with over a decade of experience and the founder of Critter Care Collective, "One Team, One Goal: Collaborative Pet Care." She is committed to making pet health information accessible and practical for all pet owners.

Dr. Chivvis is the author of The Dog Owner's Guide to Health Emergencies, a two-time Gold Award–winning book recognized for its clear, practical approach to emergency preparedness. She has also authored a children's picture book series, activity books, ABC books, and adult coloring books that combine education and creativity.

Through her books and educational resources, Dr. Chivvis works to bridge the gap between veterinary professionals and pet owners, helping families make informed decisions when health concerns arise.

✉ CritterCareCollective@gmail.com

🌐 www.CritterCareCollective.com

🌐 www.TheDVMAuthor.com

⧉ @crittercarecrew

⧉ @TheDVMAuthor

Thank You!

Thank you for choosing this guide to help you care for your cat during life's unexpected moments. I created this resource to offer clear, practical advice for health emergencies, empowering you to respond confidently with the help of veterinary professionals. I hope you found this to be a valuable read!

~Dr. Chivvis

If you found this book helpful, you might also enjoy
The Dog Owner's Guide to Health Emergencies.
That guide provides the same practical advice as this one, helping you prepare your dog for emergencies.

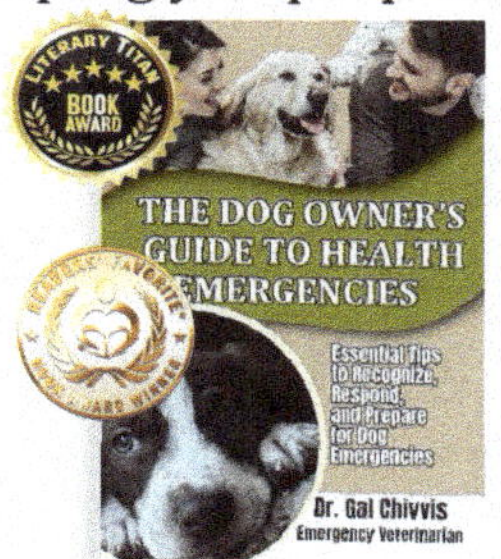

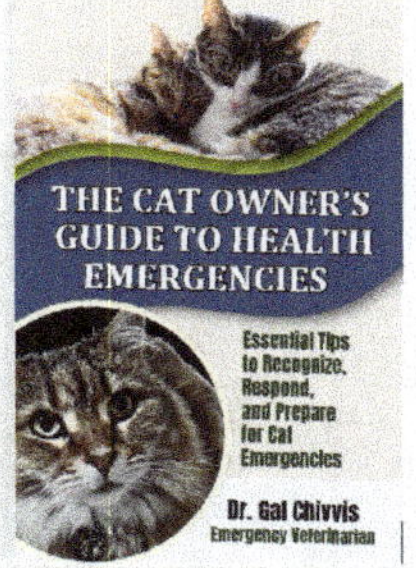

Explore more books and resources for both adults and children on my website or Amazon, including activity books, picture books, and coloring books designed to entertain and educate young minds.

Scan Here

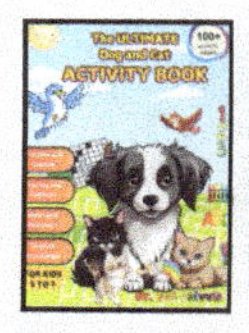 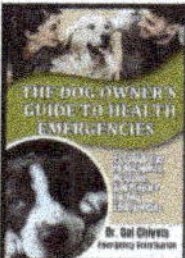 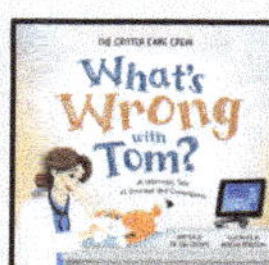 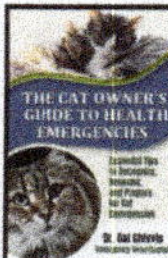 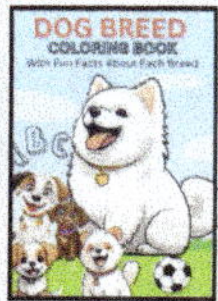

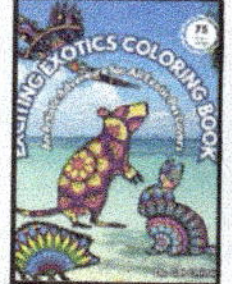 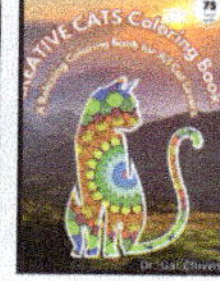 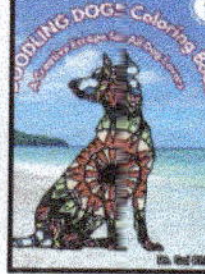 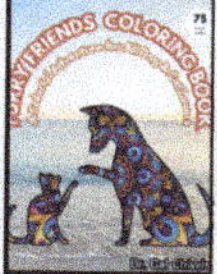 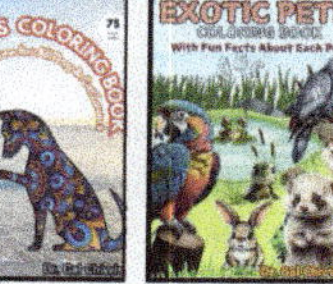 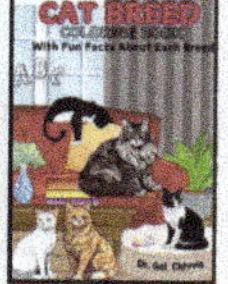

www.ingramcontent.com/pod-product-compliance
Lightning Source LLC
Chambersburg PA
CBHW071619030726
47598CB00001B/352